Mammy Diaries

MARIA MOULTON

ORIGINAL WRITING

978-1-908282-54-5

A CIP catalogue for this book is available from the National Library.

Published by Original Writing Ltd., Dublin, 2011.

Printed by Cahill Printers Limited, Dublin.

To every mam who took the time to share her story, I
only regret that I could could not print them all.

To the "Cork Mums," whose support has meant more to
me then I can ever express.

And of course, to Jimmy and the girls. Best. Team.
Ever.

Thank You. x

Contents

In The Beginning...

Gestational Airlines
Attention all passengers, this is a final boarding call for all those traveling on Gestational Airlines Flight 375 non stop service to MOTHERHOOD. At this time we would like to ask all pregnant women to proceed through security to gate one. All husbands, partners, boyfriends, significant others, friends, family and interested parties are asked to remain in the terminal building. Your flight will depart at a later time through another gate.

For safety reasons, passengers are forbidden to bring quantities of liquids greater then 100mls through security aside from those which you may be retaining.

Our flight time is an estimated forty weeks with no scheduled stopovers. Our arrival time is as yet undetermined and there is currently no data available on our destination. All fares are one way only and completely non refundable.

For those of you who experience nausea and vomiting, sick bags have been provided in the seat back in front of you. For your comfort, Gestational Airlines have also provided you with extra large seats as you can expect to gain between fifteen and forty pounds throughout the course of your voyage. These seats are fully reclinable as the journey is quite exhausting and frequent naps are greatly encouraged.

Our in flight crew are happy to assist you in any way possible, however, due to industry cutbacks, it may take some time for you to be seen to and the quality of care may be reduced.

As this is a long haul journey, we recommend that you take regular (gentle) exercise and make healthy choices from our extensive, in – house menu in order to reduce the risk of flight related complications. There will be no smoking on board the aircraft and drinks service has been suspended for the duration.

For your reading pleasure, we have provided you with a wide selection of pregnancy related literature. Please be advised that such items are for entertainment purposes only and not to be used in place of proper medical care and supervision by a trained GP or midwife.

We are also offering a special range of heartwarming movies, television programs and commercials guaranteed to tug at the heartstrings and tear ducts of all our weepy women. Headsets and tissues can be obtained from the cabin crew.

We have been informed by the captain that delays can be expected and turbulence is near unavoidable, so fasten your seat belts (loosely and not directly over the abdominal area) as we are in for a bumpy ride.

Thank you for choosing Gestational Airlines. We hope you enjoy your flight.

Chapter One

The First Trimester

Signs of Things to Come...

So, you've peed on a stick and made it turn color, CONGRATULATIONS!!!!!!!   You are now officially in your "first trimester" which depending on who you talk to is the first 12-14 weeks of your pregnancy. This is often the loooooooooonnnngest and most trying time as well as your body goes into overdrive building an entire human being from scratch. Even the most keen and eager Mary Pregnant herself will at some point find herself cursing mother nature as she awakens at one, three and five in the morning to pee, yet again....

Signs and Symptoms

Had I seriously suspected that I might have been pregnant, I probably wouldn't have taken a pregnancy test in a public toilet. For those of you considering taking such rash action, I must seriously advise against it. If it turns out to be positive, you will never live down the shame of receiving such life changing news whilst surrounded by mysterious puddles and the odor of stale urine.

So why, you ask, did I waste ten euros of my hard earned money if I was expecting to get a negative result? What strange little occurrences was I experiencing that had me reaching for the pee stick in the first place?

Well for starters, my period was late. That in itself was not a spectacular occurrence. My cycle varied from month to month, lasting anywhere from thirty one to thirty seven days. This particular month however, we had passed the magic forty day mark, which is about the time my brain emits a very loud, very shrill, warning signal, entreating me to, "get thee to a pharmacy!!!!!"

I was also feeling a bit fuzzy headed and my breasts were like two very large, very painful rocks strapped to my chest. Again though, not entirely unusual and until this point I'd passed them off as PMS. In the end, it was a bottle of wine that had me reaching for the test sticks.

I'd picked up a lovely rose for that evening but being a bit of a cautious person, I wanted to first ensure that there was no chance that my uterus had landed a tenant whose brain cells I could inadvertently be destroying.

Well, that bottle of wine turned out to be a lovely present to one of my girlfriends and the fuzzy headedness just got increasingly worse over the next nine months. As for the breasts? They reached proportions matched only in the pages of certain top shelf magazines.

And that was only the beginning.....

You see, mother nature is a very sneaky woman. She helpfully provides us with a whole range of maladies and discomforts to alert us to the possibility that we may in fact be expecting. Some of the more common symptoms are as follows:

EXHAUSTION!!!!
Holy Mother of GOD! Saying that pregnancy is tiring is like saying that jumping out of a plane without a parachute is "kind of" risky. Big understatement. I mean seriously, I have never felt such bone numbing, mind boggling, head wrecking fatigue. It was as though I was only given a few good hours each day in which to get as much done as humanly possible before completely shutting down. I woke up each morning with a six hour expiration date at which point I needed to ensure I was in the immediate vicinity of my bed as total collapse was imminent.

Do not be ashamed of your sudden inability to stay up and watch the evening news. YOU ARE GROWING A HUMAN BEING FROM SCRATCH. That takes a lot of energy. My advice? Nap loads and buy some really nice pillows and bed sheets, you'll be seeing a lot of them...

Emotional Mayhem
Holy Hormones Batman! Pregnancy wreaks serious havoc on your state of mind. You think PMS is bad? HA! Times that by about a billion and you might start to get the picture. For me, the first trimester of pregnancy was a blur. Literally. I couldn't see for the tears that seemed to constantly be filling my eyes. I cried when I was happy, cried when I was sad and god help anyone who tried to watch television with me. It got to the point where I had a roll of tissue with me at all times "just in case." Even just thinking about my perpetual state of weepiness was enough to bring on the waterworks.

When I wasn't crying, I could usually be found in the anger aisle of the hormonal supermarket that was my mind. I didn't even try to reign in my temper at work and instead gloried in my newfound ability to tell people to eff off without fear of recrimination. Nobody can get mad at the Pregnant Lady!

How my partner didn't leave me is one of mankind's greatest mysteries....

I Need to PEE
When you are pregnant, you will gain many new skills. Among these is the ability to locate every toilet within a ten mile radius. Say good bye to a solid night's sleep as you find yourself waking at one, three and five in the morning to stumble off to the toilet, yet again.....

And speaking of toilets.....

Constipation
As much time as you'll be spending in the bathroom, it probably won't be spent doing any number twos. It appears that your body's first priority now is keeping that new little life inside of you healthy and growing away. Other functions, like your digestion, will be scaled down for the duration.

Oh yeah, and whatever you do, DON"T STRAIN!!!!!! If you do, you just might end up with a nice case of.....

Piles
Seriously, just when you thought that pregnancy couldn't get anymore glamorous..... For those of you that don't know, piles - or hemorrhoids as they are properly called – are basically swollen, blood filled veins in your back passage area. They are a common occurrence during pregnancy and often caused by straining whilst constipated. Even if you don't get them during pregnancy, don't celebrate too quickly. I thought I was free and clear and often gave a smug little smile when I heard of other women's struggles with these painful, itchy demons. Better them then me! And then I gave birth... Remember that bit about straining?

Nausea
As if you weren't spending enough time in the bathroom already! It is estimated that about half of all of pregnant women experience morning sickness, which, as we all know, should be renamed "All day and All night" sickness. Nausea can rear it's ugly head at any point in your pregnancy but it's usually at it's worst in the first twelve to fourteen weeks, as are most of your pregnancy symptoms.

Changes in your Breasts
Do your boobs hang low? Um, yes as a matter of fact they do. They are also twice their normal size, hard as rocks and they HURT! If I haven't said so already, I'll say it now; hormones can be a real bitch!

Just like you, your breasts have a lot of changes to undergo as they prepare for their most important job ever, feeding your baby. In fact, these changes feel very similar to the changes a lot of women experience every month before their periods and so are often confused as PMS.

They can grow and become engorged which is really quite painful. Your nipples might tingle and at some point will darken and pretty much double in size. Veins will appear to the extent that your creamy orbs will soon resemble a road map. It is perfectly acceptable for a pregnant woman to hang a DO NOT TOUCH sign from each of her breasts during the first trimester. Of course, for some women, and their lucky partners, this increased sensitivity is a very good thing indeed.......

Really cool fact? The scent of the amniotic fluid is actually the same as your nipples. When your baby is first born, he uses this scent as a sort of primitive GPS to find his way to the breast for that all important first latch. In fact, if you place your baby on your chest immediately after birth, he'll find his way there without any help at all. It's called the breast crawl and personally, I find it pretty amazing.

Baby Brain
Have you ever lost your keys only to have them turn up three days later in the neighbors freezer? Have you ever walked into a room and then forgot why you were there? If so, then you have a vague idea of what pregnant women go through on a daily basis. Unlike most pregnancy symptoms however, this one doesn't go away when the baby gets here. It... um... I'm sorry, what was I talking about?

Missing Period
I have a big problem with those fictional women in books and movies who miss three periods and don't even notice until one day after they puke up their dinner for the twelfth day in a

row they find a tampon in the bottom of their purse and think "hmmmm....? When exactly was my last period?"

BULLSHIT!

Any self respecting, sexually active, modern woman with two brain cells to rub together who finds herself in the position of having had unprotected sex will damn sure be keeping track of whether or not Aunt Flow arrives for her monthly visit!

A Feeling.....

Okay, so it's not the most scientific method of detecting pregnancy and it's accuracy rates aren't exactly what you'd call astounding. Even so, it happens. It's the fertility equivalent of "Spidey Senses" and a lot of women swear by it. How many times have you heard a newly pregnant woman claim that she, "just knew" even before she took the test?

Of course, the fact that she was throwing up her meals, falling asleep at the cinema and hadn't had a period in four months might have had something to do with it as well...

A Positive Pregnancy test

Signs and symptoms are all well and good, but most, if not all of the early signs of pregnancy can – maddeningly - also be symptoms of PMS. At the end of the day, taking a pregnancy test is the best way of determining whether you are or aren't pregnant. Now, let me be the first to say, "Congratulations."

Real Mams Talk About:
How did you know you were Pregnant?
Not only did I pee on a stick, my husband got it as part of his birthday pressie! I Knew I was Pregnant as I had tender breasts, had to go pee during the night and was like a bee-atch! Always a sure sign for me.

With my first son I remember looking at this line on a stick and even though I knew I was pregnant (that old adage about you "just knowing" is so true!) I couldn't believe it. It was a bit of a shock to be honest as I had been "chemically controlled" for the best part of a decade and fully expected my body to take six months or more to co-operate. Hah! With my second boy, again, I knew I was pregnant before I even took the test. That was just a confirmation really. But that time round I knew my optimum dates to conceive and made good use of them!

Gwen, Kildare,

Well we had decided the previous month to try for a baby so me being me, I went all out and read up on charting temps and cervical mucus and I signed up with www.fertilityfriend.com to keep track. It told me when I should expect to ovulate so after, when my temperature stayed high I had a tiny feeling. Then I really started having symptoms, like really sore, hard boobs and I took an instant dislike to coffee, which I had always loved! I thought it would take a while to conceive so I bought a ten pack of tests on ebay plus a First Response for the proper test. One morning in early October, I decided to try a test to see how it worked and I saw the very faintest pink line. It was so faint you really had to squint to see it but I tried again the next morning and it had got stronger. That's when I went for the First Response and it was positive too!

Ingrid, 29, Cavan

To be honest I didn't know I was pregnant. Myself and my husband had been trying to get pregnant for three years. I could have sold shares in pregnancy tests! I had been on clomid for five months and was doing yet another test when that glorious second line popped up! After that, I took another, ummmmm… six or seven tests, just to be sure. Sad and all as it is, I actually have one of the tests in her baby box.

Leanne, 26, Donegal

Both times (pregnant twice) I missed a period. First time I was trying to get pregnant so I was very aware of everything. I'd been doing my morning basal temperature for six weeks to see when I ovulated in my cycle. I'd heard stories of how hard it was to get pregnant so I thought it might take awhile and hey presto, a few weeks after deciding to try, I was! I had very regular cycles so was late by three days by the time I did a test (as though putting it off would really make sure that I was? Really logical I know! NOT!) So I'd bought the tester the night before and waited till the next morning as though my pee would be somehow stronger first thing in morning to give a 'good' reading. I'd always written down when I got my periods and when I was due all my life, a habit my Mom got me into for some reason. I know many women who don't so when they say they're trying for a baby, I always encourage them to start that habit. When I look back, the time before I missed my period, I was unnaturally tired and I cried a lot the weekend before (hormones!)

The second time around we'd just been 'thinking' about having another baby and I had just finished my period that day so for some reason thought I'd be okay! I know! In hindsight, another daft notion but at the time!!! It was my seventh anniversary too!! Anyway, my anniversary present that year came nine months later much to our delight and she was born at home. We went on holiday a week or so later (from conception) and I thought the sea air was just knocking me out and that I had bad PMT but when I got home and was late, I did the test and the rest is history.

Samantha, 34, Laois

I took five tests but only three were positive... Strange that, as my period was nine days late. The only reason I though I might be pregnant was that I had a very unusual amount of wind.. (too much info?)

Ciara, 33, Dublin

I think I knew the week after I got pregnant! The first thing was that I went off my beloved smokes completely, couldn't understand why I wasn't enjoying them! The the next weird symptom was an eye twitch that just wouldn't go away. I had it for about five weeks!! It was horrendous and no matter how much sleep I got, it would never go away. I would spend hours researching it on the Internet, self diagnosing. Then there was the tiredness and the need to eat everything and anything I could lay my hands on. I did about five tests all together as I knew I was pregnant before I missed my period, so they came back negative at first but I was convinced I was and then the day that my period was due it came up as positive.

Maria, 25, Dublin

When I got pregnant, I knew within the first week. I couldn't drink my glass of red wine one night (which was amazing for me!) I felt extremely tired and even had a midday nap, which again was so not like me! So the earliest that they say you can do a test, I did, and the first drop of wee that hit it made the pregnant sign practically jump off of the stick! I never did another test because that one was so strong that I had no doubts. Also, the morning I did the test, I had that really strong metallic taste in my mouth. I just knew it!

Jane, 32, Dublin

Finding Out: Kathy's Story

I was mortified going in to buy the test. I don't know why because I've been married for three years. I guess it was more the "I know what you've been up to! Ha ha ha..." feeling. Then, when I got to the counter, I barely got the blink of an eye! Then there was the decision of when to take the test. So I drove home and went into the toilet while my husband was tidying his car and took the test. I didn't have to wait, it just turned blue straight away. Yep! Definitely pregnant. Oh. Okay. What do I do now?

I walked out of the toilet as my hubby was coming in with his tools and what have you, "Oh, by the way," I heard myself say, "I'm pregnant." (That's not exactly how I imagined telling my husband if we were ever to get pregnant.)

"What?" he asked, " How do you know ?"

" I just took a test"

"Why?"

" Because I had a feeling."

"Oh. Right. Let's see the test. Oh, right, grand. Now, where is that screw driver?"

End of conversation.

Was this how it was supposed to go?

Kathy, 32, Louth

Real Mams Talk About:
Finding out...

I honesty cannot repeat my reaction to finding out I was pregnant the first time, but once I was about fourteen weeks, I got really excited. Needless to say, he was not planned quite so soon! As for my partner, well, considering that he had just handed in his notice to his work the week before and had no job to go back to... When I told him the news, he asked me to go and get some logs for the fire. I took the hint and left for thirty minutes. By the time I got back, he was delighted, if still a little shocked. With our second (who was very planned!) he was thrilled, although a little disappointed as I had only come off the pill in December and was pregnant by January. He was hoping it would take a few months of "trying!!"

Christine, 29, Wicklow

We still had those, "Oh crap. Are we crazy?" thoughts when we found out, but overall, we were delighted. We were apprehensive too, as we had previously had two miscarriages and knew that anything could happen and nothing was certain.

Jennifer, 33, Dublin

We had been trying for three years, so you can't plan anymore than that! We were in total shock for quite a while. We were absolutely over the moon at the thought of being parents.

Leanne, 26, Donegal

Because I kind of knew that I was, I had already thought things through. On seeing the positive pregnancy test though, my emotions still got the better of me! It was unplanned but within seconds I just knew it was the right time. My partner was on the phone to me as I took the test. On reading the result my first words to him were, "Congratulations daddy." I swear, there was the longest pause ever! Hearing myself say the words made it all the more real and I threw up with sheer emotion. He was shocked but delighted.

Kim, 22, Dublin

Myself and my partner made the decision to start trying while on holiday in July. I came off the pill and six weeks later, I was pregnant. I was scared, happy, excited and worried about how his family would take the news. The day I told him, he was driving me to work. I was quiet on the drive, as even though we'd decided to do it, I was a bit worried he had really only agreed for me. When I told him, he said nothing, just kissed me as I got out of the car to go into work. I was worried at this point, but then, twenty minutes later, I got a text saying he was shocked but happy and we would be okay.

Mam of Two, Monaghan

When Two become Four...
What was your reaction to finding out you were going to be the mother of multiples?
Shock and disbelief! Actually sometimes I still don't believe it! I went to the EPU for an early scan, suspecting I had or was going to miscarry. I had been obsessively doing pregnancy tests and was worried that the line was not getting stronger. The sonographer was not too happy that my GP had referred me as I was only six weeks and she said we may not see a heartbeat and then I would be more anxious. She had the screen turned towards her and was taking ages. I really was expecting her to say there is nothing there. "Well", she said. "I've got something to tell you and its not what you were expecting" She turned the screen around and there were two heartbeats banging away. I can't actually remember what I said. I just remember saying to her later no one will believe me. I went home in a daze, bursting to tell someone but found the house empty and had to wait for my husband to come home. When he same in I said Sit down, I've news. Straight away he said its twins isn't it? We honestly didn't know whether to laugh or cry, I think I was laughing manically for a while!

Emer, 35, Mayo

I nearly died when I found out I was pregnant full stop, never mind lying there being scanned only to be told that basically I was pregnant twice! I didn't believe what he was telling me just like I didn't believe what the pregnancy test had told me several weeks before... I have to be honest and say I really thought my life was over, and from that moment I think I actually blocked it out.

Niamh, 30, Roscommon

I had been with my partner twelve years and we'd been in our house for three years when we decided to try for a baby. We were twenty months trying. Eventually, after relaxing and not trying so hard, we conceived. I was eight weeks when I found out and at twelve weeks had a bit of a show and straight away thought I was miscarrying. I went into the emergency room at the hospital. They did a vaginal scan and there was the baby moving away like no one's business. I was delighted. The doctor then said, " Ah look! The other one is asleep!" I couldn't believe it. I said, "Sorry?" she said, "You're having twins!" I was overwhelmed as I thought I was losing one, only to find out there was an extra one in there. It was brilliant. I called my partner in and told him. He couldn't believe it. We were delighted. We rang all the family. I think we just laughed for the next few weeks. it was brilliant

Elaine, 32, Dublin

I cried with emotion. I couldn't believe it. I felt so special and was dying to get out of that room to ring everybody wanted to shout it from the rooftops. Such a great feeling it was over whelming

Amanda, 36, Meath

The Fear
Oh God, I am freaking out. I know, I know, I'm pregnant and growing an entire human being from scratch inside of my uterus, which until now has pretty much had as much responsibility as a self cleaning oven that has never been turned on, let alone baked anything. How do I even know that it's going

to work? That it's going to know what to do? How do I know that it won't burn the biscuits?

It's not fair. In every other aspect of my life, I have some semblance of control. I see the results of my efforts on a regular basis. But this, the most important project of my entire life, is completely out of my hands.

I have become addicted to those websites that tell you what is going on with your baby and your body, week by week. I know when he or she is growing fingernails, when his or her "tail" -blech- is going to turn into legs and that by the time I go for my first scan, my little one will be a whopping three inches long.

I know that it is normal to feel as though I've been hit by a truck and to fall asleep in the middle of the evening news. I know that waking up to pee five times a night is to be expected and that according to my mom it is Nature's way of preparing me for all those sleepless nights ahead. I know that crying during the Angelus is a result of hormones and that I'm not actually being moved by the spirit.
I also know that about one in five pregnancies end in miscarriage and that not all babies are born healthy and well.

This scares me. I want there to be some sort of guarantee, a way of knowing that everything is going to be alright. I wish there was a contract I could sign, a promise that if I take my vitamins, eat healthily and don't smoke, drink or take drugs that everything will turn out just fine. I want to know for sure that these pains they say are normal are really just my ligaments stretching and not mother Nature's way of letting me know that I am one of the unlucky ones.

I can't wait until I'm further along, until I'm out of this stupid "first twelve weeks" crap. I want to go for my scan and have the doctor say that everything looks fine. I want to be able to see my baby on that little screen and know that there are two arms and two legs and that everything appears to be normal. I want to know that this is real and that it's not just a big mix up, that the lines on the pregnancy test were right and that my period isn't just really, really, late.

I want my baby to be okay.

A Scare

I was just about nine weeks pregnant on my first baby when I had a tiny bit of spotting. Up until that point, even though I'd known I was pregnant, I didn't really KNOW I was pregnant, if you know what I mean. Despite the positive pregnancy tests and the visit to the doctor, I had yet to feel that connection with the little person growing away inside of me.

I didn't look pregnant, I couldn't feel my baby moving, in fact, if it wasn't for the insane mood swings that had my poor partner fearing for his life and my new found ability to pee like the proverbial racehorse, nothing had really changed. And then I saw the blood....

There wasn't much of it, just a few pinky brown streaks like the start of a period, but it was enough to send terror coursing through every vein in my body. I spent the night crying my eyes out, terrified I had lost this little being who until now I'd had no idea how much I loved. My world shrank smaller and smaller until there was just me, my womb and the little person inside of it. I prayed and I cried and I begged God to let my baby live. My partner held me close, telling me that everything would be all right. Finally, I slept.

The next morning, I calmly dressed and called a taxi. I had no tears left to cry – or so I thought – and when I arrived at the hospital, I walked to the information desk, opened my mouth, and bawled my heart out.

The Midwives couldn't have been nicer. They took me straight to emergency and explained my situation to the women there as I was in no position to speak for myself. They helped me fill out the forms and someone stayed with me until I was called to the scan room. I lay on the table and prepared myself for the worse. The Ultrasound Technician was lovely. She placed the wand on my abdomen and a moment later she smiled and turned the screen to face me. There, bold as brass, was my baby's heartbeat, thump, thump, thumping away.

The tears, which had finally stopped, started again. This time though, they were tears of joy as I realized my baby was still there. That we still had a chance.

First Pics

I had to wait until I was twenty weeks pregnant to get a scan in the hospital (Semi Private.) I couldn't wait to see If I actually had a baby inside me or if I was just crazy! At this stage I wasn't showing and I had been feeling so shit that I really was starting to think I was just mad.

I was getting angrier and angrier with the length of time that I had to wait. It is hard waiting. And then I had loads of worries, what if I was pregnant and there was something wrong with the baby? Had I done anything that might harm it?

Well, the scan day finally came. I brought my mam along as my husband had just got a new job and I didn't want him to have to ask for time off so soon. He was okay with this. As he said himself, "sure, it's all women's business anyway."

I was bursting to pee when I got to the hospital and popped into the nearest toilet and oh god, the state of it! There was toilet roll up the wall and everything! This was in the public part and I'm not really that fussy but this was bad.

Panic set in. I couldn't do this. I should have forked out the thousands for private care. I can't handle this. I went out to my mam, she calmed me down and we headed over to the semi private area. What a difference! Why is it not like this for everyone? Women in Ireland should protest more, demand more.

Anyway back to the scan. The midwife was very matter of fact. She was showing a student how to do the scan, so while I mostly got to see both of their elbows, my mam got to see everything. I went into over drive with questions like, is the heart beating okay? Does it have legs? Is it okay? How is the Nuchal fold?... Thankfully, everything checked out okay.

I didn't ask about the sex as it makes no difference to me. My husband wants a boy so he agreed that we should just leave it and not find out. I thought I'd cry when I saw the little image that was printed out, but I didn't and I got annoyed with myself. What was wrong with me? Had I no heart?

Mam was all emotional about it, but I was just glad everything was okay. I went over for the bloods and to see the consultant. The Midwife sped through loads of questions. Thank god mam was there, as I was lost and couldn't hear her properly. I went into a panic that I might have Aids or Hep C and whatever else they were testing me for. I didn't want to know about all that horrible stuff.

Then she said I'd have to have a glucose test at twenty eight weeks for diabetes because of my weight. Again more panic, I'm still waiting for this test and still worried about it even though I have only put on two pounds. When I got home I showed my husband the scan. He smiled. At last, I thought, some recognition.

"What is it, did you find out?"

"No, I didn't want to know, it's healthy and I'm happy." I replied.

He smiled.

"Thats good."

Kathy, 32, Louth

Real Mams Talk About:
The First Scan...

This was at about twelve weeks. It was so strange driving to the hospital about to see the reality of why I was feeling the way I was. Until then it was just a concept, and surreal. But even seeing the little baby on the screen didn't change that. I was in denial throughout the pregnancy. Feeling disconnected from what was going on. The photos were brilliant though, really clear. Amazing one of the hands. The miracle of creation, that even at twelve weeks and three centimeters long, this person was developing inside of me. We didn't find out the sex, to us it was like unwrapping a gift before Christmas. And, as someone said, we don't get a lot of surprises in this life so why find out? And also, why find out in order to know what color clothes to buy or what color to decorate the nursery? Such banal decisions.

Chris, 31, Cork

My first scan was at ten weeks. We were so worried as I'd started to bleed. I was afraid to look at the monitor then I heard my consultant say 'we are still in business' and looked up to see my little baby. It looked like he was waving at us. We didn't find out the sex of our baby at that time. It was at the twenty week scan when we asked.

Josephine, Cork

My first scan was a nightmare! We waited our turn in the waiting room and when we finally got in to see the ob, he popped me up on the table. Good god! The excitement of seeing it was overwhelming. He searched and searched for ages but couldn't find anything. Our hearts sank. We were sent to another part of the hospital for an internal. We had to wait another three hours to have this done. It was the longest three hours of my life. When we were finally seen, the nurse did the internal scan and there it was, all tucked up right at the back where the doctor couldn't pick it up. The relief was unreal. We didn't find out the sex – it ruins the surprise.

Leanne, 26, Donegal

We had our first scan at eleven weeks. There were arms and legs flying everywhere! Well, two years later and nothings changed there! We were on a high. It was a bit weird to think that this wriggler was in there growing and moving and I couldn't feel anything. We never wanted to know the sex of the baby, but painted the baby room blue and everyone thought we had found out. I have a scan scheduled this Wednesday for numero two. I'll be 9wks and 3 days ish. I'm Looking forward to it. Dad and I keep having day-mares that we'll told there's another one in there!

Niamh, 35, Louth

The first scan was so amazing. Even though I was going public, I went for all my scans privately as the earliest I could get them done in the hospital was at twenty weeks. When I went for my first scan, I thought I was twelve weeks but the baby was actually dating fourteen weeks and three days and it was just so amazing. Afterwards, myself and my boyfriend went for breakfast. I looked at the picture and just cried. It seemed so real and it just made my heart melt. I was in love. I didn't find out the sex but at a scan at thirty eight weeks to check if the baby was still breech, I saw a Willy and balls and told my boyfriend that I thought it was going to be a boy. I was right, even though up until that point I was totally convinced that I was having a girl!

Maria, 25, Dublin

Real Mams Talk About:
The Best and Worst of the First Trimester...
The best part was finding out I was pregnant. The worst... Have
you got a pen? The list is long; I was wrecked. I just wanted
to curl up in bed and sleep for the full nine months. I was a
bit depressed - maybe this was the tiredness? - and I wouldn't
get out of bed. I couldn't eat, I only wanted oranges and soup
(yuck, when I see that written down!) I had very bad headaches
but wouldn't take anything in case I damaged the baby. I didn't
have morning sickness but I may as well have as I felt awful and
looked awful too. My husband got fed up with me being in bed
all the time. He thought I was putting it on. The women in his
family didn't act like this, what was wrong with me?

I thought about losing the baby all the time and how I would
be very mature about it if it happened (yeah right.) I thought I
was mad and made the whole pregnancy thing up, maybe the
doctor and the test were wrong. I thought about all the bad
things that could be wrong with the baby. What if it had a
learning difficulty etc... I worried about what kind of parents
we would make. My husband wasn't saying much so I worried
about what he was thinking. I worried about our relationship.
I worried about finances, I worried about where I lived, I worried that I worried too much and that I was affecting the baby
and so on it goes... I had good thoughts about the baby, how it
would look, its personality, playing with it feeding it, dressing
it, watching it. But I suppressed these thoughts, just in case.
Well, it happens to so many women, why would I be the lucky
one to be allowed to have this baby?

Kathy, 32, Louth

The worst first! My mood changes dramatically. I'm argumen-
tative, moody, tired and tend to feel hungover! If it was possible
I would like to spend this time in a tent in the middle of a field
and have someone drop by with small meals three times a day.
Do not expect me to talk to you though! I NEED MY SPACE –
both physically and mentally. The best? I Suppose it's knowing

that you're pregnant. It's lovely having this secret all to yourself before you tell anyone. It's really and truly your time with the baby. Once you spill the beans about your bean, you're public property! You and your bodily functions!

Gwen, Kildare

The worst thing for me with both my pregnancies was the tiredness. No one prepared me for just how tired I would be. I was heading to bed at 8:30 most evenings. I also hated the greasy hair syndrome! I adored the feeling of being pregnant, that there was a little life growing inside me, and that as my husband is adopted, I was carrying the only blood relatives that he would know. I couldn't wait to get a bump!

Christine, 29, Wicklow

The worst was definitely the fear that I might have a miscarriage. I had signed up with rollercoaster.ie and found it great for making friends and getting tons of advice and support. However, each day I logged on it seemed that someone else had lost their baby and I dreaded that happening to me. The best part was the feeling that I was growing this new life inside of me. I would look up pictures and information on which nut or fruit my baby resembled in size each week. I also loved the special secret feeling I had especially in work. I'd be sitting in a meeting with my hands on my tummy under the table, off in another world. The baby was on my mind 24/7 for the entire pregnancy.

Ingrid, 29, Cavan

Exhaustion, there is nothing like it! Also the Queasy turns, in particular, one sixteen hour vomit-a-thon which was the result of not taking it easy enough. The headaches were terrible too. I haven't had anything as bad this time around, I'm probably just used to being permanently knackered! I Hope the headaches don't start though. They were the worst. Also, it was quite tough dealing with the weight gain and trying to cover it up, even though most likely it wasn't really obvious at all.

Anne, 35, Louth

The best aspects were the little secret we were carrying around and the tenderness, gentleness and excitement that my husband showed to me. The worst bits were the tiredness, nausea, lack of appetite and hating cooking for my husband as well as the stress of constantly making up excuses for the way I was feeling. Oh, and the increase in boob size even at an early stage. I was happy with my little boobs and to suddenly have them start to swell was not good!

Chris, 31, Cork

Chapter Two

THE SECOND TRIMESTER

Notes from a Tiny Tenant

My belly is jumping. I am hiding in my living room while my baby sleeps in the bedroom, quietly watching the show being performed by the tiny acrobat who has taken up residence in my body.

Biff! Boom! Zap! Pow! I wish I had those spinning signs from the old Batman show. I'd make them appear every time the tiny babs splashed out into his or her daily workout routine.

This little one is a lot more active then the snot queen was when she was on the inside and I can't help but wonder - with more then a small amount of guilt - if it's the new baby's way of saying "I'm here! Notice me!" A premature bout of sibling rivalry, if you may, a taste of what's to come.

There's no denying that this pregnancy has been a completely different experience to my last go round. Last time, it was all brand new and I had all the time in the world to obsess over every last detail of my pregnancy and the little life that was growing within. I was that most revered of creatures, the first time mum.

I would spend hours lying about feeling my baby move and imagining the watery world they inhabited. I religiously did my kick counts and labored for MONTHS over what would be included in my birth plan. I signed up for pregnancy yoga as soon as I was able and stopped work at six months so that I could thoroughly relax and enjoy every second of the experience.

I worried about every move I made and how it could possibly effect my child. I took notice of every tiny kick and swirl she made, and if more then a few hours passed without my feeling her, a panic greater then anything I'd ever known would consume me and I'd rush to lie down until she started her dancing again. For nine months my world shrank to a tiny little bubble - population two.

This time around, the bubble is a little bigger and my days are spent running around after the soon to be big sis, watching with wonder the seemingly endless stream of milestones she accomplishes. Seeing her go from sitting to crawling to pulling herself up to standing. I am in awe of her abilities and of the tiny clock that only she is aware of that tells her when it's time to learn something new. I could sit and listen to her chatter for hours. She amazes me.

So involved am I in her little world that I often forget about the watery world that exists inside of me and the tiny tenant who inhabits it.

And then there are moments like now when with a single, solid kick, my big, round belly leaps to the side and I am reminded once again of the little person within. A person who is not their big sister and who may very well come out not baldy and fair but with a thick head of dark hair. A person with a mind and personality of their own. A small little someone who one day soon will come out into the world and change the dynamics of all our lives, forever.

For now though, all is quiet, and for the moment at least, my world has once again shrunk to the tiniest of islands - population two.

Real Mams Talk About:
The First Movements
The only word that comes to mind is magical. You know that
there is a baby in there but when you feel the baby move, it
becomes so much more real. The movements start early apparently, but I only felt them from about four and a half months
onwards. Straight away I made the husband feel. He would sit
for ages with his hand on my tummy, waiting for them.

Anna

On my first pregnancy, I had no idea what to look for. I didn't
know what to expect. In the end, it was rather like gas bubbles
and I didn't really notice them until I was about twenty two
weeks along. In hindsight, I 'd probably been feeling them for
a while and passing them off as wind! On my second baby, I felt
it much earlier, around sixteen weeks. My poor husband had
such a hard time of it. It seemed every time he came near me,
the little ones held their breath and went very, very, still. When
I was around twenty six weeks, we bought one of those heartbeat listener things so he could hear the baby that way, even if
the little rug rats were playing statues!

Donna, 36, Roscommon

I'm a bit hazy on the first pregnancy but I think it was around
sixteen weeks. On the second pregnancy it was definitely quite
early, around twelve weeks at a Christy Moore concert! I rec-
ognized the movement from before, probably missed it first
time around! My hubby said he saw the movements before feeling them so it was well into the pregnancies, probably around
twenty weeks. The were fluttery to begin with and more defined
as the baby moved. The babies seemed to roll across your belly
at times as they shifted position.

Samantha, 34, Laois

I can remember watching Home & Away and feeling three tiny
little tap, tap, taps just under my rib cage with my first son. I
have no idea however, how far gone I was. With my second son,

I was in bed one night reading at twelve weeks. I Felt a flutter but I ignored it as I thought it was much too early, even though it was my second pregnancy. I felt it again the following night. And the next. It was then I knew that my dates were right and the doctors were wrong! It wasn't until twenty two weeks that my husband felt the first kick.

Gwen

I think I started to feel movement at around fourteen weeks, but being my first I didn't know for sure. I remember my dad saying of course I'd know, but how could I? I'd never done this before!

Caragh, 30, Cork

Ann Summers Maternity and Nursing Wear
Dear Ann Summers,
I had the pleasure of being invited to one of your parties last night and must say that I thoroughly enjoyed myself! Being almost 38 weeks pregnant, I particularly enjoyed perusing your maternity line which, by the way, you do not advertise heavily enough at all!!!! Therefore, I have taken it upon myself to promote a few of your more "mom friendly" items.

. The "Mia Baby-doll, String Set and Tickle Ties" was the first item which caught my eye! With it's open front design allowing room for your expanding belly, this charming number can be worn all through pregnancy and beyond! It's front tie ribbon closure is both charming and practical as it allows easy access for nursing and the ribbon tie underpants make for easy undressing in those later days of the third trimester when bending over can be so uncomfortable!

My one complaint (and this seems to be a common thread throughout your maternity wear by the way!) is that the woman modeling the outfit must only have been in the very early days of pregnancy as she was quite tiny which made it very tricky for me to identify this as "maternity wear" Perhaps in future you could use women a little further along then "the morning after?"

I must commend you though on including the "Tickle Ties," as not many outfits come with toys for the baby! These fluffy little fiends will provide hours of amusement for your small one although I wouldn't recommend leaving them to play with them unsupervised as both the feathers and ribbons offer a choking and strangulation hazard. Oh well! Points for trying:)

."Pipa Crotchless Skirt" Now this item was a real charmer! I don't know why Mothercare hasn't brought out a line of these yet! Once again, I almost missed this little gem as a part of your maternity collection but upon closer inspection was able to distinguish it for what it really was...

For those women who wish to retain a little bit of modesty and femininity while in labour, the "Pipa Crotchless Skirt" is definitely for you! With it's frilly black skirt keeping your front bits protected from prying eyes and it's attached crotchless panty allowing the doctor or Midwife easy access to your exposed vagina, you can forget about worrying over the state of your pubic area and concentrate instead on bringing your new little life into the world! What more could the discerning "Lady in Labour" wish for?

I would however, suggest a small re-naming though in order to grab a larger portion of the "expecting" market. Perhaps the "Peek a Boo Modesty Maternity Skirt" would be slightly more appropriate.

. In that same line, I also found what is perhaps one of my FAVOURITE items! The "Pippa Baby-doll and string set." This nursing nightie is both stunning to behold with it's slinky black baby-doll design with pink satin trim AND it's remarkably practical with it's cutaway "peek a boo" holes which completely reveal the nipple and full areola for breastfeeding ease! Again, a rename may be in order, but with the proper marketing, this could easily become a best seller!

. Regrettably, I would have to advise parents against shopping in your "Toy" section as many of your items, whilst made of child safe, medical grade rubbers and plastics, also contain small parts which could pose a choking hazard and your "edible" selections may provide hours of fun, but are entirely too high in sugar for my liking! Kudos though on the use of body parts not commonly seen in children's play items. Highly educational and extremely pioneering, although again, some of the colors and sizes may not be anatomically correct representations and therefore confusing to small minds.

. Your commitment to breastfeeding is to be applauded even if your methods are slightly misguided. The nipples will eventually toughen up by the continual suckling of your infant, additional assistance by use of nipple clamps is unnecessary and may actually put the mother at a higher risk for blocked ducts and mastitis as well as causing unnecessary pain and discomfort.

Your selection of nipple care products is quite extensive and while I understand that some of them may have "cross market appeal" you may want to rethink the labeling on some of your gels and lotions as their names can be quite misleading! As well, while many people may be under the impression that a baby may be enticed to drink more if mother's nipples tasted of strawberries, chocolate and Pina colada, studies have shown that this is not the case. Also, the high levels of sugar in these products can have a detrimental effect on your baby's oral health.

I was quite charmed by the large range of products available for babies in the breech position. Studies have again shown that babies in the womb are sensitive to noises and sensations from the outside world and these vibrating wands, when placed against the tummy, will gently encourage your small one to turn into the proper birthing position, thus reducing the chances of a

Cesarean Birth, the rates of which have soared in recent years! Your use of phallic design as a symbol of fertility also brings into play the male essence which was necessary in the creation of this little life and lets dad feel more a part of the process. Your "Rabbit" line is sure to give older children a giggle and let them become more involved in your pregnancy and welcoming their new little sibling to the world as well!

I'm afraid I must comment yet again though on the need for better labeling as there is a great need for such an innovative product as this and a lot of women are missing out on something which could potentially (and literally!) turn their pregnancy around.

Overall Ann, I have to commend you on your commitment to pregnant and nursing mothers and making them feel good about themselves during such an important part of their lives. However, I do feel that without proper labeling and marketing, sales in these areas are doomed to fail and threaten the viability of your entire maternity line (if it hasn't already!)

If you would like any help with this, I am more then happy to offer my skills and services and maybe together, we can "turn things around."

Yours Sincerely,
Maria xxx

Real Mams Talk About.....
Maternity Clothes!
We could not afford maternity clothes with my first son, so I wore most of my normal clothing and would cut into the elastic of my track pants to accommodate my growing belly. With my pregnancy now, I have vowed that I will definitely get maternity clothes as I think they make you feel pretty.

Anna

I tried to avoid them for as long as possible and instead bought bigger sizes which was just a disaster as they make you look bigger in every way. When I started on the maternity clothes at twenty two weeks, I went to Top Shop, desperate to cling on to "me" and my long gone youth. Some comments I got were that I looked a lot neater, but maybe that's just sympathy votes! This time I think I'll just bite the bullet and go with mammy clothes as soon as I have to. Boo Hoo!!!

Catriona, 35, Louth

I got lots from friends and then I bought some nice, special stuff to make myself at least look better than I felt. Every night before bed, I set out what I was going to wear the next day and that would make me feel nice. I think it's important to not jump straight into a tracksuit. Of course, towards the end they are great. I was two weeks over with my son so they were great in the evenings to relax about in.

Fiona, 28, Kildare

When I started to show first, I used to leave my top jeans button open and hold them up with a hair bobbin looped around the button! I couldn't wait to get into Maternity clothes though. One day in work (before I told them) I had a maternity top on and my boss was showing me something at my desk. After, I went to the loo and noticed that the tag was sticking out plain as day with, "Maternity Wear" wrote on it! He definitely had to see it!

Ingrid, 29, Cavan

Maternity Clothes are awful, there is such a lack of choice. Finding a bra to fit me is impossible, I have been measured three times and each time I have been given the wrong size. It was either too big, completely non supportive, or else too tight, making one big tit! I ended up with a bra that covered my whole chest area and more and made my boobs look droopy, so I have gone back to my normal bras and yes, I know that you're not supposed to wear under-wire, but I am. I got a few nice t-shirts in Mothercare and two nice pairs of jeans from Oxendales. A wedding outfit for my brothers wedding was hard to find. I found a lovely non maternity dress in the end. I think I'm a bit glowing now, I'm more relaxed about pregnancy.

Kathy, 32, Louth

I wear my own clothes as long as I can, usually till about five months at a push. It annoys me how the neck line of maternity tops is always cut very wide and low, but maternity bras are generally full cup with wide straps, so your bra peeks out a lot. The range available is much better these days.

Lara, 28, Meath

God! What a nightmare! Well, I'm big anyway, so to find them in larger sizes was so hard. I found a few and then kind of lived in them, ha ha! I didn't socialize much while I was pregnant so thankfully didn't have to shop for anything fancy! Some of my friends literally bought an entire new wardrobe full of maternity clothes which I think is just stupid. All you need are a few pairs of maternity jeans, trousers and tops. Tops were easier to buy as lots of the styles were flowy and so you just bought your usual size or one up. I much preferred spending my money on my new arrival than on ugly maternity clothes..

Sam, 27, Wicklow

It's a ......WHAT?!?!?!?

A friend of mine - who is also heavily pregnant - recently found out that she is having a girl. Her news got me thinking...

Ever since we discovered we were expecting for the second time, I've just assumed that we would have another girl. I have it in my head that I am meant to be the mother of girl babies, that I have some sort of "lady gene" which prohibits me from producing a male until I've popped out at least three of the fairer sex.

Take my family history for example; my mom? Three girls, then two boys. My Uncle? Three girls, one boy. It just seems that if you start with a girl, you go on to collect the entire set before adding a boy to the mix, at which point you realize that they are a whole new set of troubles and stop procreating altogether. Add to that the fact that we have enough pink, flowery clothing to dress at least ten baby girls simultaneously and you can see why I find the thought of having a boy rather perplexing...

Obviously I don't care what we have so long as the child is healthy and well, but to be honest, I really don't know what we'd DO with a boy! (and by we I mean me as I've a feeling my partner would be more then comfortable with a little more testosterone around the place)

For starters, I am more then a little freaked out at the thought of the penis and all it entails. When I was visiting home last summer, I had the experience of watching my sister change her son's nappy. Being the mother of a young baby myself, I considered myself expert in such matters. Even so, I got the shock of my LIFE when she took off his nappy. WHAT THE HELL WAS THAT?!?!? Obviously it was his penis and yes, as my child's conception was far from immaculate I am fully aware of the physical differences between males and females, but still... my baby doesn't have one of those.

This brought up a whole new set of questions. How do you clean it? How do you keep them covering the place in pee when they're having "air time" (nappy free time for those of you not in the know) I assume it produces somewhat of a sprinkler effect. With little girls, it just sort of trickles out onto the towel beneath them.

I suppose I'd just have to consult the expert on such matters, his father, who, by the way, dealt quite admirably with the delicate flaps and folds of our girl child when first confronted with one of her messier creations.

Also, boys seem to be that bit more "rambunctious" then girls. Having observed the social interactions of my friends' babies, I no longer give any truck to that whole "It's how you raise them..." crap. As far as I'm concerned, in this area at least, Nature kicks Nurture's ASS! They're mad little creatures, full of vim and vigor from the get go. While the girls are happy to take regular "sit breaks" where they happily sit and play away, the little men are like freakin' action heros in training! They NEVER STOP MOVING!!!!

It's a bit of a shock to the system to be honest, to think that somehow, with my lifetime's experience of all things pink, soft and estrogen fueled, my body could create a little person who will grow up to be broad, hairy and more then likely, his dad being who he is, a devotee of the cinematic offerings of Sylvester Stallone.

But for now, my little princess is stirring from her nap and needs changing and dressing for the day. It's sunny and warm outside, I was thinking maybe something pink.
Only time will tell.

(Author's Note: HA HA HA HA HA HA HA HA HA HA HA HA HA HA HA HA HA HA HA HA HA HA HA HA HA Oh the Naivete! My darling daughter number two was born shortly after the writing of this piece and to put it mildly, the child is a lunatic. Willy or no willy!)

Antenatal Classes: Gwen's Story

My husband and I went on a day long antenatal class when I was expecting my first son. It was really enjoyable, but then, I'm the type of person who enjoyed her pre - marital course as well! To be quite frank though, it all went out the window when the time arrived as I was induced and was very much, "Okay, you're the professionals here!" And, "That sounds fine. Whatever you say!"

I suppose they're helpful enough for your first pregnancy but you could tell them a thing or two yourself the next time round!

My second birth was a totally different experience due to all the reading and research I did into the type of birth I wanted. I was also much more confident in my body's ability to do its job. In fact, thinking back, the classes can be extremely negative for first timers!

With my second son, I read up on and practiced hypno - birth-ing which was absolutely wonderful! I read all the positive birth stories I could get my hands on and bombarded the birth/labour forums on line for advice. There are some wonderful women on there with such good advice to give!

I kind of got roped into attending the classes second time round and when I was asked by the very friendly midwife giving them, what was I doing there as I had done all of this before, I was quite honest in replying that it was a perfect excuse to get out of the house on a Tuesday night for an hour or two.

Gwen, Mother of Two plus one on the way, Kildare

Real Mams Talk About:
Antenatal Classes

Yep, I did a prenatal class. It was fun as well as informative. I remember the Person who ran the course telling us about the build up to the birth and taking a bath. She then asked, "and what will you put in the bath?" To which a mum shouted out, "whisssssskey!" We were all doubled over laughing. And just in case anyone might be tempted to put whiskey in the bath, lavender oil was the correct answer (boring, I know.) Jokes aside though, I would definitely recommend doing one as it was a great help.

Luke's Mom, Cork

I went to a private one at around thirty four weeks. It was good as I knew nothing about birth other than books I read and Internet forums. It cost fifty euros for a one to one session and was well worth it for me anyhow. We put a nappy on a doll and gave it a bath. I wouldn't have known how to put a nappy on my baby otherwise!

Laura, 30, Cork

Due to an unprecedented number of women due to give birth the same month as me, I was unable to get into an antenatal class that would finish before my baby was due, so I missed the classes that discussed the actual birth. The Internet told me all I needed to know!

Lara, 28, Meath

They were okay, I run a lot and they warned against running, especially on the treadmill. When I asked my doctor why, he said it was in case I fell off. They were a little over the top, naive and catered for the totally clueless ... in my humble opinion.

Ciara, 33, Dublin

I went to prenatal classes and never went back after the second class. She didn't tell me anything I didn't already know, except about the size of an epidural needle!

Leanne, 26, Donegal

The classes were useful only because I discovered all the hospital policies and what they 'wanted to do to you,' i.e, breaking waters, internals, episiotomies (like it's just slicing a loaf of bread not layers of your precious body!!! Ugh. I went home and re-wrote my extensive and over the top birth plan to include in bold type everything I didn't want done, which they seemed to do as a matter of course! The woman from the La Leche League was sweet but trying to illustrate with a doll in front of men and women, most of whom have probably never seen anyone breastfeed in real life, was laughable! As for the birth video, it was outdated, old fashioned and unrealistic! The whole experience was out of date!!! A decent documentary would've been more useful.

Samantha, 34, Laois

I did both a course of public ones over a couple of weeks as well as a six hour private session for eighty euro. All were fantastic. People who don't do them are pure mad! I ate the pregnancy books and was addicted to rollercoaster (Irish parenting site.) I searched the Internet for more and more information. Knowledge is definitely power! I swear, there were a couple of people who were also pregnant behind me in work and I was the guru! I'd love to offer antenatal classes and am gonna look into it when I get a spare second, in about twenty years!

Orla, 34, Limerick

Hypnobirth
When I was pregnant on my first baby, I remember hearing about something called "Hypno Birthing." Like many things in my life, I immediately got a picture in my head and formed an entirely wrong opinion about the subject.

I imagined all sorts of things, from someone swinging a giant watch whilst muttering away about being "very sleepy" to roomfuls of women with dopey looking smiles completely unaware that a human being was sprouting from between their legs. Oh, and obviously these make believe women all had names like Rain and Moonbeam, grew their own clothes and lived in edible houses. Needless to say, my views on the topic were more then a little bit skewed...

It wasn't until I began the research for this book that I started to question myself as more and more women were sending in their birth stories saying that they had had a hypno birth. Then, something happened which I had not previously forecast. I was contacted by Miss. Hypno - birth Ireland herself (she prefers to be called Tracy) inviting me to a weekend seminar. Oh. My. God. I nearly wet myself with the excitement of it all.

My partner, being as knowledgeable and open minded on the subject as myself, was not exactly open to the idea at the start, but quickly gave in after being blasted with a good ol' dose of what I like to call, "Crazy Pregnant Lady."

So in we shuffled, bracing ourselves for an onslaught of in-cense, love and whale sounds, only to be met by a tiny, neat looking woman in khaki trousers and a pinstriped shirt. The room itself was filled with five or six average looking pregnant couples chilling out on beanbags and drinking tea.

I was so confused! Where were the chimes? The mind alter-ing incense? More to the point, WHERE WAS THE GIANT WATCH?!?!?!? These people just looked like everyday, run of the mill pregnant people and Tracy looked more like a school teacher then the 1960's style "Guru" I had envisioned. It was about this point that I began to realize that I may have been a teensy bit wrong about just what hypno - birthing entailed...

GentleBirth, by Tracy Donegan

Stack the deck in your favor of having a positive birth for you, your partner and your baby. You've heard the scary stories that everyone is hell bent on telling you. You're wondering if there is anything you can do to give yourself the better chance of a normal birth, a birth that where you feel calm, confident and in control ? That way is the GentleBirth way.

If you think hypno - birthing is only for hippies, read on. Most couples come to GentleBirth workshops not because they are completely ruling out the epidural but because they want to do everything they can to have a positive experience for themselves *and their baby* with or without an epidural.

They understand the reality of our overstretched, overstressed maternity system and want to learn how to navigate their way confidently and calmly. GentleBirth mums are women from all walks of life - teachers, stay at home mums, solicitors, scientists, midwives and students. Like you, they've all heard the scary stories and have decided to stack the deck in their favor of having a great birth experience rather than leaving the biggest day of their lives (and their baby's) to chance.

GentleBirth is about reinforcing the choice we have as parents to determine how our children are brought into this world - that choice, that responsibility, doesn't start with labour--it begins now.

GentleBirth is the only birth preparation class of it's kind in Ireland. The workshop is for parents who want to be actively involved in decision making and prefer to have an understanding of what choices are available to enable them to make informed decisions confidently.

Is your partner prepared for labour?

Dad's have a huge role in labour and are very eager to understand what they can do to help. During the workshop you and your partner develop a clear understanding of how to navigate the overstretched, busy Irish maternity system confidently and calmly. Dads/birth partners appreciate the importance of their role as birth supporter, facilitator and advocate on this very special day.

GentleBirth antenatal weekend workshops combine birth hypnosis (deep relaxation for pregnancy and labour) and active birthing principles enabling couples to have empowered, confident birth experiences with or without medical intervention at home or at the hospital.
Although labour and birth is a serious topic the workshop is a lot of fun (and nobody goes home barking like a dog!) There's plenty of practice too, so it makes for a very relaxing, informative weekend.

Over the weekend parents to be learn the following and more:

Physiology of the normal birth process

Fear Vs Relaxation in Labour - keeping adrenaline at bay

The application of sports psychology and mental training for birth

Neuroscience for birth - rewiring your brain from fear to confidence

Facilitating the perfect balance of hormones in labour - undisturbed birth

Breath awareness during labour

Comfort measures for labour and birth (what you and your partner can do at each stage)

Use of the birth ball and other tools in labour (including water birth)

Bonding with your baby before birth

Routine procedures in Irish hospitals and how to avoid unnecessary labour interruptions

What happens on admission to hospital?

Becoming a calm, confident birth partner

Creating an effective birth plan and how to communicate your intentions and preferences

Informed decision making

Relaxation techniques for mums and partners for pregnancy and labour

Why you don't have to push!

Birth positions

Breastfeeding

Recovery tips

Turning a breech baby - the use of moxa and hypnosis.

Participants also receive a GentleBirth guide, three practice CDs for Mum, a free Confidence Builder download for Dad and handouts. Mums and Dads are also invited to join the GentleBirth yahoo chat group and connect with over two hundred other excited GentleBirth mums around Ireland.

During the workshop you will meet other couples who also want to have an active role in working towards a very positive experience. It gives you and your partner a great opportunity to escape life's day to day demands and just focus on each other and your baby for a weekend. Couples leave the workshop feeling excited about labour – a lot less anxious and ready for the great adventure of parenting - now immune to the scary stories everyone can't wait to tell you!

For more information on GentleBirth courses, visit http://www. GentleBirth.ie The five week GentleBirth Homestudy course is also available for mums unable to attend a workshop.

Tracy Donegan is a mum herself, student midwife, breast-feeding counselor and Elected Chair of Our Lady of Lourdes Maternity Consumer Group. Tracy is a regular contributor to Modern Mum pregnancy magazine and Infant & Child Magazine and has been featured on RTE's Baby on Board and 21st Century Child. Tracy is the author of an informational guide to childbirth options in Ireland (The Better Birth Book) as well as "The Irish Caesarian and VBAC Guide."

Chapter Three

THE THIRD TRIMESTER

"I went overdue on all my 3 kids, so the last week always involved having strange aches and pains and me constantly wondering whether this was start of something soon. its kinda scary but exciting at same time."

Mary Kelly

Three for a Tenner

Oh God. The reality of this pregnancy is finally starting to sink in. In just over twelve weeks (TWELVE WEEKS!!!!!) the new baby is going to be here. TWELVE WEEKS!!!! Where the hell did the time go? Doesn't this baby know that it's not due until the start of June? And doesn't this same baby know that June is FOREVER away?

June is summer. For the kids and teachers it marks the beginning of summer holidays and the end of the school year. In order to get to June, you must first pass lent and Easter. It was the sun that did it you know. So long as it was rainy and miserable and dark, June was as far away as my toes now seem most most days. And then something happened....

Without my really noticing, the cold and miserableness slowly disappeared and a lovely warm breeze swept in. A news item about baby lambs on RTE declared Spring to be here. Instead of two layers of shirts and a puffy winter jacket, I was now able to bring my daughter for a walk in a nice light hoodie (still wearing her hat and blanket mind you!) The days started staying lighter just a little bit longer and then, the ultimate sign that winter was on the way out...Tesco started stocking Easter Eggs. Boxes and boxes of brightly colored chocolate eggs, their foil wrappers begging to be unfurled, revealing the chocolatey goodness within...

How did it happen? I still have days when I forget that I'm even pregnant! Which, if you could see the size of my bump these days would show you the depth of my delusion. My last pregnancy crawled by. It lasted FOREVER!!!! This one seems like it's barely started and already I'm approaching the finishing line.

Back up the boat! I have things to do, places to go, people to see.... The book isn't finished yet, I still need a publisher (if anyone knows of anyone in the bookworm, wink wink, nudge nudge...) We are due to move house in a month, we don't know where we're moving, the freezer door still needs fixing and I still haven't gotten the courage to tell my landlords I lost my keys!

Last week, everything was okay. Last week, we had until the baby got here, we had until June to finish off our to do list. This week though, this week is a different story altogether, because this week, Tesco's is stocking Easter eggs and June is twelve weeks away.

Oh well, at the moment, they're still full price. When they're marked down three for a tenner, that's when I'll start to panic...

One of those Days
It's official. I'm all used up. The well has run dry. There's no room at the inn and whatever other metaphors you can think of for being completely and utterly worn out. Even my typing skills are failing me. So far, in this paragraph alone, I've had to correct about ten different typos already (ironically enough, I misspelled typos as tpos and had to go back and fix it.)

Maybe it's the giant baby I'm growing inside of me that is now resting deeeeeeep within my pelvis causing me to pee a little every time I sneeze. Maybe it's the hips that seize up every time I walk more then five steps. It could be the teething baby who has rediscovered her love of my "empty since the stick turned blue" breasts and has made dry suckling into an art form. Maybe it's waking up with said baby at five a.m yesterday morning and again today at four.

Then of course there's the apartment that seems to dirty itself every time I turn my back and the seemingly endless list of things to do before we move into our dream house. The drunks that line the river and try and reach into my buggy every time I walk past definitely don't help matters. Nor does the ridiculous amount of dog poo that people feel free to leave in the footpaths which inevitably ends up on the wheels of the buggy.

Mix into all of this the guilt that I feel when I snap at my partner or feel as though I'm being less then the perfect mother and partner (bullshit I know, but hey, you try controlling your emotions when you're seven months pregnant and then get back to me) and that constant battle between wanting to do more and knowing that if I even try to add another item to the list, my already stretched sanity will snap completely and everything will come tumbling down.

It just seems as though all of my time is taken up doing the the things I have to and that as hard as I try, there never seems to be enough time for the things I want to. Or maybe today's just one of those days...

Reality Check
I've been such a moaner later. I've actually managed to irritate myself this last week with my feelings of "Woe is me" and general end of pregnancy crankiness. I desperately needed a knock round the side of the head and yesterday got one in the form of the loveliest text from a good friend who recently had her second child.

I had texted her with the intention of (what else?) having a quick moan about wanting the baby to get out NOW and let me get back to normal life, to being able to walk comfortably and sneeze without wetting myself etc... and so asked her how she had managed to get through the last weeks of her pregnancy. Her reply reminded me of all the good things I was forgetting about being pregnant:

Feeling the kicks, pokes and rolls of this small person you've never met but have grown inside of you for the last nine months. This is the last time you will experience that sort of closeness with them. Once they're out, they're everyone's, but for now it's just us...

Looking GORGEOUS while pregnant. I don't care how vain this sounds, but I never feel as sexy, attractive or womanly in real life as I do when I'm pregnant. Even my clothes fit better! Although that being said, it will be nice to expand my clothing options beyond "whatever stretches over the belly!"

The way that most people seem to love a pregnant woman and smile when they see me coming. I love the excitement that a new life gives even to perfect strangers. That and the fact that people feel obliged to be extra nice to you and let you sit down and eat loads of biscuits and such...

. This is the last time that we will be a family of three. The time between now and the new baby's arrival is the last time that Lily will have our full, undivided attention. I think about the way our days are now structured around her and her needs. I think about our morning cuddles and lazy days spent pottering about together. That's all about to change for her and there's no way to explain it, just do our best to enjoy these last moments and hope that when the time comes, we will have the patience and time to remember that she still needs us too...

As I read her reply, I added another one silently in my head as I thought about all the couples who would love to be in our shoes but for reasons of biology or reasons unknown are unable to conceive a child or else have great difficulties in doing so. I think as well about the families who have lost children and the unbelievable pain and suffering they've had to endure.

I know how incredibly lucky and blessed we are to have our gorgeous, healthy daughter (snotty as she may be at times) and to be expecting number two any day now and if I have to wait just a little longer for that moment, then I'll grin and bear the aching joints and embarrassing "mishaps."

As a good friend of mine told me last time around, " When the fruit is ripe, it will fall."

Real Mams Talk About...
Things you will miss about being pregnant, and things that you won't!
I won't miss maternity clothes, the extreme tiredness, the waiting or the lack of energy. I guess I'll miss my old life a little. When he was a bump I still had my freedom and now I'm suddenly a grown up and its a bit sad even though I love him and he is a little ball of giggles. Sometimes I am a little jealous of my friends .

Fiona, 28, Kildare

The only thing I missed was the feeling of babs moving inside. Everything else was pretty hideous and I had it really easy!!! So there's the reality. Who are these nuts who say they loved being pregnant? You get no sleep, NO SEX, swollen everything, you have strange dreams when you do get five minutes of sleep and you feel like you'd eat your left arm if people weren't looking at you and wondering if you're having twins, triplets or quads and you only six months gone! I swear to God, I'm a teacher and the kids just couldn't get over the size of my bump. Rumors abounded of twins and waters breaking in class... And here we go again!

Kay, 35, Louth

I loved that people let me sit down, opened doors and chatted to me about when I was due. I felt very special. I looked forward to a glass of wine, a cold beer, opening buttons on my trousers (all my maternity ones were elasticated) getting back to running and fitting into my dressy clothes again!

Ciara, 33, Dublin

I will not miss the heartburn or the piles, the nausea, the restless legs, the inability to sleep for more than two hours at a time and not being able to eat and drink what I want. I will miss the constant attention from my husband and my little son kissing my belly and asking when is his baby coming out!

Lara, 28, Meath

I will not miss SPD, Peeing every two minutes, busy bodies with their useless advice, sleepless nights, and strangers touching my bump! I do miss those wonderful moments when the baby kicks and I also miss my bump actually, it made a handy shelf for propping up books and cups of tea and I spent all day just rubbing it.

Ingrid

Oh, where do I start? I won't miss the tiredness, the constant trips to the bathroom, the mission to put on socks and shoes, the sickness and definitely not the backache! I will actually miss the bump. After carrying it around for the best part of a year, it becomes a part of you in a way. Feeling the baby's movements were such special moments and once it's gone you realize how much they meant to you. I also will miss how nice people are to pregnant women.

Kim, 22, Dublin

I loved all of it, well okay then, maybe not the tiredness, but that is about it. I do miss the bump, even though I have a beautiful baby, I got kind of used to the bump...

Christine, 29, Wicklow

I definitely won't miss the insomnia, the heartburn, those sharp pelvic pains you get when you stand up, the breathlessness and not being able to give my babies a proper cuddle on my knee. I will miss that mad feeling that you only get once you are no longer pregnant and you see a pregnant person and suddenly feel that little bit jealous wishing that you were there again (even though it was such an uncomfortable experience.) I blame mother nature. It's her sneaky little way of making us keep the species alive!

Jennifer, 33, Dublin

The bad moods. Feeling like an elephant. Heartburn. The constant weeing!!!!!!! The painful kicks. (I know!!!!) Being uncomfortable at night and not being able to roll over with ease! That uncomfortable "full" feeling all the time! I'm looking forward to being a bit more agile, breastfeeding and believe it or not, getting pregnant again! I want to be able to drive without there being two people behind the steering wheel!!! Oh, and have the ability to get in and out of the car without making small children stop to take a look and have a laugh at the fat lady!

Gwen, Kildare

What I miss about being pregnant is being proud of my belly, and feeling my baby kick, tiny little ones at first then big moves. While I was pregnant I spoke to my baby all the time. After the birth I had no one with me in the shower to talk to. I missed that.

Luke's Mom, Cork

Perineal Massage
There is a lovely activity called "Perineal Massage" which involves oiling and massaging the perineum - otherwise known as the patch of skin located between your vagina and your anus - in an attempt to increase it's elasticity so as to avoid tearing during childbirth. For those of you giggling in the back, this is not the time for girlish modesty. That ship has long since sailed...

Now, I don't know about you, but this is not an area that I want to be taking any chances with. The word "episiotomy" makes me queasy and when I hear terms like first, second and (ugh) third degree being bandied about in relation to damage done in the areas down below, I want to curl up in a ball and disappear to a far off land where babies really are delivered by stork.

However, a few awkward sessions involving me, my less then spacious bathroom, a bottle of olive oil and some contortionist work that wouldn't have been out of place in a circus ring, had me questioning the whole process and wondering if there wasn't another more, umm... pleasurable manner of tickling my fancy...

For the record, two babies and one very happy husband later, my bits remain intact.

Real Mams Talk About:
Perineal Massage
Yes I did! On the first baby I did everything known to woman-kind to ensure I didn't have an episiotomy. My sister had one on her first baby four months previous to the birth of mine. She was of the opinion that the less you knew about the whole thing the better. I was the polar opposite.
I found it hard to do as the bump was in the way. I don't even know if it worked except to say that I had only the slightest of tears and no stitches. The perennial massage, as it's known, is very uncomfortable and bordering on painful and I didn't bother on the second baby. It's something you want to do in privacy and my two and a half year old didn't let me pee alone, never mind put her through watching me do that!
Samantha, 34, Laois

Yeah, tried that, for all of two seconds. Just too gross (sorry) and I tried every other hint and tip under the sun. Just decided to let whatever would be happen, and guess what? I had an episiotomy cos my baby was just not going to move with out the help of the old salad tongs (forceps.) So no thanks to the fanny massaging this time around!

Louise, 34, Waterford

I believe I just blushed............I really would not know!!!!

Anna

Didn't try it, thank God! I'm with you on the lots of sex bit. My sex drive went through the roof while I was pregnant, so that was definitely a better way of doing it!

Leanne, 26, Donegal

Ummm... yeah... did that massage alright. In fact, it wasn't me who actually did it, it was the hubby! But I only started asking him to do it about two weeks before so I don't think it was enough cos I had to get an episiotomy.

Jane, 32, Dublin

At the prenatal class we were advised to buy a bottle of sweet almond oil and rub it on the perineal area after every pee. Of course I always ran to the loo, only to find I'd forgotten my oil. So much peeing to do, so little time to be organized. I ended up having a bottle in every toilet in the house. As to whether it worked or not – I ended up having a caesarian, so I don't really know.

Luke's Mom, Cork

I didn't try it. Massaging down below (assuming I could reach around my huge belly!) is not something that appeals to me. If I wasn't so tired, I would probably try the second technique, however, that isn't happening too often these days!

Lara, 28, Meath

Tried but failed cos I couldn't reach it!!!

Laura, 30, Cork

And since we're in the area and (kind of) on the topic...

Real mams Talk About...
Sex and Pregnancy
My sex drive rocketed during pregnancy. Couldn't get enough...
like the giant chocolate buttons.

Leanne, 26, Donegal

Sex? What's that??!! Ours were assisted reproduction babies,
so a lot of the romance had gone from our sex life before the
kids arrived!! We try, we really do, but exhaustion usually takes
over.

A, 33, Dublin

In the first trimester and half way through the second, I was
too tired for anything, but then I turned into a randy b*tch and
would wake my husband up at various stages through out the
night!

Christine, 29, Wicklow

Well sex . . . .whats that ??? Ha,ha sorry, l shouldn't laugh but
to be honest we're only now getting back into it. We never 'did'
it the whole time l was pregnant and then I had a third degree
tear so we only 'tried' to do it a couple of months after our baby
was born but it was absolute agony for me. It's only now in the
last few weeks that we've started up again. We talked about
it and hubby said watching the birth actually put him off . . .
he said watching babs coming out of there put him off coming
near me. Not sure if thats a normal thing for men ?? He's grand
now though.

Ruth, 36, Dublin

Mine definitely increased on both pregnancies and this time he
only has to look at me, feels mad...

Elaine, 29, Cork (Expecting no. 3)

I still enjoy sex, but am just too tired sometimes. I keep thinking that it may never be the same again so I'm getting as much
as possible in now (which is not much either!) I'm not really

interested in getting the big O, so sex has been relegated to quickies with no complaints from my darling husband!

Kathy, 32, Louth

I reckon there are two types of "duty" sex, neither of which are enjoyable. The first is pro-creation sex, so clinical. And the second is induction sex. Again, so clinical and uncomfortable. We tried the induction type with our first son (once!!) and it was so horrible we said never again!

Gwen

Up, down, up, down, up, down... That's not the mattress by the way! Mad for it, repulsed, wasn't getting any anyways as it might poke baby in the head! And before you laugh, yes, he's got a HUGE one! To make matters worse, the guy next door and his then current bit of fluff were like dogs in heat and all I can say is that she must have been an opera singer!!! OoooooooHHHHHH MYYYYYYY Goddddddddd!!!!!

Emma, 27, Kildare

I lost all interest in sex but also it was physically impossible due to my SPD. My partner was very understanding and it was never an issue. He is a saint!

Ingrid, 29, Cavan

My sex drive wasn't affected the first time around. The second time, sex was on my mind all the time! This time it's trying to get time on our own. Just when you think you have time for a quickie, in strolls our daughter like she knows we're up to something!

Monaghan Mama, 32

Nesting

Do you know how much you can accomplish when you get up at five in the morning? I didn't, and had no intention on ever finding out until this morning, when, having gone to bed at eight pm, instead of her usual "somewhere in the wee hours" my little sweet pea awoke after nine solid hours of sleep and declared herself open for business.

I on the other hand, had, true to form, stayed up until past midnight reading - of all things - a book on infant sleep - and was in no mood to have my slumber disturbed for at LEAST another three hours.

Alas, it was not to be and after forty five futile minutes spent trying to convince the princess that yes, she really was still sleepy, I caved and rolled bleary eyed into the kitchen to prepare breakfast for the infant overlord, now busy squeezing out poos on the potty. Charming.

Daddy meanwhile, slept on.

Seriously, how do men do it? I have yet to decide if they simply do not hear the wailing infant six centimeters away from their ear or if they blithely choose to ignore it, confident that mammy will take care of everything. Thus allowing them to sink back into sweet, sweet slumber. I am afraid to think too closely on this one for fear of my reaction. I do still need him to pay the bills after all...

Anyhoo... Poos done and breakfast eaten - hers, not mine - my little angel proceeded to pull herself to standing by the bookcase and happily set about emptying every shelf within her reach. I, on the other hand, was feeling the ever present "nesting" instinct kicking into high gear and suddenly seeing dirt sprouting before my very eyes.

I started in the kitchen. Telling myself to keep it in check, I tried to satisfy myself with simply wiping down the counters and brushing the floor. But like the addict I've become, it wasn't enough. I needed more. I moved onto the stove, scrubbing the range and getting the bits of dirt out from under the dials and soaking the bottom of the oven in baking soda and water. From there it was a small step to putting in a fresh load of laundry (or two) and folding that which was already dry. When I noticed the dust in the fireplace, my eyes lit up with the zealousness of the true fanatic!

At this point, I put on the kettle for a cup of tea only to realize that brushing the floor hadn't quite done the job and instead used the boiling water to mop the floors in the kitchen, sitting room, hallway and bathroom which I then vacuumed for good measure...

By the time my partner roused himself at half past eight, our house had been scrubbed and sterilized from top to bottom and I was a sweating wreck in the sitting room, our daughter gazing at me warily from her perch by the (spotless) coffee table. By nine, the fervor had dimmed and it was back to bed for a well earned nap. By the time most people were beginning their day's work, my to do list had long been cleared!

We are moving house in a month's time. As I scan the rent ads each day, my brain is already moving ahead to the next challenge, packing up our belongings for the big move. It's like Christmas come early... I can hardly wait.

Real Mams Talk About:
Nesting....
I had a toothbrush out at times, scrubbing, mowing lawns, planting flowers, cracking the whip to get wall papering and painting and carpet cleaning done. I think it started seriously about six weeks before D - Day.

Louise, 35, Louth

The last few weeks I cleaned CONSTANTLY. Even though the rooms were spotless , I still could not stop cleaning and sorting the baby things. My other half thought it was hilarious!

Kim, 22, Dublin

Oh my god! I cleaned and tidied like never before. I could see dirt everywhere.

Fiona, 28, Kildare

I got in and cleaned out my hot press and kitchen presses before the SPD took full hold. I also re-homed the four lizards I had in my living room as I decided one day that it wasn't clean enough to bring home a new born baby to!

Ingrid, 29, Cavan

With my first, we were in a small apartment, and I cleaned cupboards, windows, carpets and anything else that I could. With my second, we were in our own house, and I decided four weeks before I was due, to get the builders in to knock down walls that I had been wanting to do for three years. Once they had finished, I went into Manic cleaning mode, and landed myself in hospital with a placenta tear! My advice ? Nest, but not manically!

Christine, 29, Wicklow

I literally tore my house apart. I cleaned all the presses, the windows , you name it and I cleaned it! I even tidied out the garden shed! My partner can't wait for that to happen again.

Elaine, 29, Cork

I bought five hundred euros worth of bedlinen in one swoop to Arnotts.

Ciara, 33, Dublin

Chapter Four

BIRTH STORIES: PART ONE

"Even talking about it now brings me to tears. When I finally delivered him I was shocked and exhausted more than anything and my eyes were closed and I just cried my eyes out I was so overwhelmed. Then they announced he was a boy and placed him on my chest. That moment alone was by far the best thing I've ever experienced and I'd go through it all again to feel that..."

Kim, 22, Dublin

Sonia's Story

The alarm was set for seven a.m. I was thirty eight weeks pregnant with twins and I honestly didn't think that I would still be waiting to have them. I started feeling a bit strange at about midnight and decided to try and get some sleep, just in case this was it. The pains however, continued, so I went to wake my husband, whose response was:

" Its only three thirty..."
"Yeah..."
"But the alarm isn't set to go off until seven..."
"WELL I'll JUST GO AHEAD AND HAVE THE BABIES ON THE FLOOR THEN WILL I?!?!"

That got his attention.

He shot out of bed and rang for a taxi. This of course, was after he took a shower, did his hair and rifled through his collection of two hundred T- shirts to find a suitable one to wear.

The taxi arrived and I kissed my sweet two year old goodbye. He was fast asleep, and I welled up, thinking, he has no idea what is about to happen to his idyllic little life. The next time he sees me I will have two other little beings to take care of and he won't ever have me all to himself again.

It was the middle of the night and the roads were quiet. The traffic lights however, were in perfect working order, and their favorite color was red. We stopped at every one of them.

This was not good as for quite some time now – since before we'd left the house actually - I'd had a funny feeling down below and could only hope that there wasn't a hand or a head sticking out! The feeling increased as we drove, to the point that I could only sit sideways with one bum cheek on the seat.

There was a garda car in front of us. Nick and the taxi driver were joking between themselves, "Oh, do you think we should flag them over and ask for an escort to the hospital?"

My darling husband, without turning round to look or indeed ask how I was doing, said, " huh huh, don't think there's any need for that now in all fairness!" and continued on with the party in the front. I, on the other hand, concentrated hard on not giving birth in the taxi. I prayed we would make it to the hospital in time.

We finally arrived. We were brought to an office to wait while the nurse went and fetched my chart. I took it upon myself to go into the adjoining changing room and put on my nightie, dressing gown and slippers. Of course when the nurse came back, the first thing she said was, " Ooh, there was no need to get changed, but if you feel more comfortable..."

I felt like a right tit and promptly turned as red as my brand new slippers!

On our way to the labour ward, my waters broke and gushed all over the floor. I gasped at the sensation and the noise of it.

I realized then that this was what that "bulging out" feeling in the cab had been and was why I couldn't sit down properly.

We continued on - with me now walking like John Wayne - and stood outside of a door waiting for the midwife. All the time I was dripping all over the floor with my clothes stuck to me, smiling hopefully at each nurse who came and went.

Eventually, someone came for us and I squelched on in, leaving amniotic footprints behind me. Our lovely German midwife told me to get on the bed. I asked her if I could get changed first . It was then that she looked at the pool I was standing in and exclaimed, "Have your waters gone??!!"

Well, duh! Hadn't anyone told her?

She fetched me a lovely hospital gown and asked if I wanted pain relief. Yes, indeed I did!!! She went to fetch the gas and air for me to use while she organized an epidural. When she came back however, her hands were empty. She said that her boss was going to examine me first.

I had just gotten my gas when the senior midwife came in, whipped up my gown and announced that I was ten centimeters dilated. She was just going to pop out for a second and when she came back we would start pushing.

"WHAT!!!!!!!!!!!!!????????????"

She came back a minute later with three other people in tow. I was taking a shot of the gas and air for the shock. The mouth-piece fell on the floor and the boss said, " Just leave it, there'll be no need for it at this stage!"

And with that she stretched me apart with her hand. I yelped with the pain. "Okay!" She said cheerily, "chin on your chest and push...."

"WHAT!!!!!!!!??????"

I just kept thinking, how is this happening so fast?   I wanted
to give your one a swift kick in the head because her stretching move was the most excruciating part of everything so far!
Instead, I just did what I was told and after about three pushes
, at 5:07 a.m, my beautiful little Mia was born. I had to look
down to make sure because I didn't even feel it! I would have
loved them to hand her to me but she was whipped away to be
checked - which I believe is normal with multiple births.

I still had another baby to deliver, so I was allowed a little rest
and a drink. When the pushing began again, it was a little
longer and a little more painful. I thought that who ever had a
hold of my right leg was about to rip it clean off. It was pulled
so far back it was almost touching my ear lobe!

Then, seventeen minutes later at 5:25am, my darling little man
Sam was out (and yes, I did feel that!)

I was quite stunned when it was all over. I felt very strange. I
was lying there looking at my two babies but it had happened
so fast that I couldn't quite take it in. It wasn't until they were
handed to me that I realized they were actually mine. I bonded
immediately. Forty five minutes had passed since I had arrived
at the hospital. I was sitting there with tea, a custard cream, two
beautiful babies and not a stitch in sight. Marvelous! Imagine
had we waited for the alarm?

Anne-Marie's Story

It all started on a Thursday morning, two weeks before my due date. I got up at nine a.m to go to the loo and noticed little puddles of clear fluid forming around my feet. I phoned my husband to let him know that there was something beginning and he came straight home from work. We took our time and made sure we had everything we wanted packed and ready to go.

We went into the hospital at about three thirty that afternoon and I was seen in the emergency room. I was pleasantly surprised that I didn't have to get an internal exam but disappointed that I was scheduled for an induction the following morning. I asked for more time to allow labour to develop unaided but I was refused at this point.

We went to our favorite Japanese restaurant and I got the hottest chili dish I could tolerate. Afterwards, we went to the beach near our home and we walked for an hour and a half. I found it hard to settle down and sleep as I was getting quite excited and expecting to feel something start at any minute. At about four a.m, I noticed that I was getting some very gentle tightenings. I put on my hypnobirthing Cd's and spent most of the night listening to them - with a bit of Enya thrown in for good measure!

We went to the hospital for ten a.m. I explained to the mid-wife that we were hoping to have a natural birth and that we wanted to wait for my labour to begin on its own. Did I have to be induced seeing as I was having some tightenings?

She spoke to the Doctor who then went and checked it with the senior Doctor. He came and spoke to me afterward and said that as I would most likely go into labour myself, I was absolutely right to wait if that was my desire. He then wished us the best of luck. I was delighted. They did however inform us that I would be induced the following morning at six if I hadn't begun to labour myself.

I was shown to the ward where I was fed like a prize goose throughout the day. We were given lots of space by the staff, many of whom had heard of and were encouraging of hypno-birthing. At nine pm we were informed that my husband would have to leave as visiting hours were up.

I felt things were definitely moving along for me and I was shocked that my husband wouldn't be able to stay with me throughout this experience. After speaking with our midwife she explained that the only way for them to know whether I was in labour or not was to do an internal exam which they would not do as they preferred to let women labour naturally in their own time.

As impressed as we were at hearing this we still had an issue of being separated. The midwife had a think about it and came back to us, she suggested that if we walked around the hospital my husband would not be in the way of the other women on the ward. She said we could do this for an hour or so and then she would run a bath for me which he could be there for also and we could see how things were going at that point.

We walked and walked every inch of the hospital. Throughout the day, the tightenings had strengthened and I had little des-ignated resting points along our circuit; chairs, window ledges, radiators, etc...

I got into the bath at about half eleven and it was glorious. Within a very short time, proper surges began. I was brought back to the ward and had the one and only internal exam of my labour. I was three to four centimeters dilated and the baby's head was still quite high up with some waters in front.

At this point the midwife said that the birth was still quite far off and that I may not even give birth that night. They phoned the delivery ward but they were extremely busy so I was told I may have to birth in the ward which they said would be fine and for me not to worry as it wouldn't make any difference to me.

I could really feel the surges intensify and although I felt very calm and in control, I was starting to find this transition difficult to manage pain wise. I was given some gas and air which did help somewhat but I found it a little difficult to manage my breathing.

I was wheeled to the delivery suite in a rush. There were quite a few obscenities en route I'm disappointed to say. When I got on the bed the Doctor said she could see the head and that it wouldn't be long before our baby would be with us. We asked that I not be cut, that I would prefer to tear if that needed to happen at all. The Doctor said she wouldn't dream of cutting.

On the second push the baby's head came halfway out, I was encouraged to continue pushing after that surge ended which I did not do. Instead, I waited for the next surge to bear down again and two surges later our baby was laying on my belly latched firmly to my breast. The Doctor checked me afterward and I had no tears so no there was no need for any stitches. All those months of perineal massage had paid off!

The period between the internal exam to the babies head appearing was very short, less than ten minutes in total. It just felt like one long, very intense surge which brought me from three or four, all the way to ten centimeters and carried the baby right down the birth canal. Really, this was the only discomfort I experienced throughout the birth.

I was delighted with how we were treated by the staff and was surprised at how hypnobirth friendly they were. I was certainly allowed to have the labour we had chosen with the full support and encouragement of the team there.

Our journey through our first pregnancy and birth have been wonderful, learning about hypno-birthing and planning a birth that we were comfortable with was positively empowering and to have our beautiful baby girl at the end of it all is just magical. I enjoyed every minute of the journey and am adoring every inch of motherhood even more.

Theresa's Story

My contractions were two minutes apart and I was three centimeters dilated when I got to hospital. I went on the gas and air then and stayed standing and moving for as long as I was allowed. I'll be staying upright and swaying my hips a lot longer this time if I can, as sitting on the bed was sooo uncomfortable!

Pressure in my back passage was strong. I didn't have pethidine, thank god. I asked for an epidural quite early on as I was afraid that I wouldn't be able to cope, but I'm very glad that I couldn't have one. I just breathed through it with the help of gas and air.

I went off into cuckoo land, thought all sorts of weird and wonderful things. I didn't talk to anyone, had my eyes closed through the whole thing and just used hand signals for more drinks, thumbs up, etc... There was nothing to distract me from dealing with contractions.

Pushing began. What a weird and wonderful sensation, like having a huge poo or orgasm, or both together if you like, no messing. I was so glad to be able to have felt that as the epidural would have killed the feeling.

As far as the urge to push? Well, get as many pushes as you can out of that pushing urge. Keep pushing and it'll take on a life of its own and will push for you nearly. I was trying to get three per pushing contraction. But after two hours of hard work, Babs was not moving. I knew things were not great as everyone stopped encouraging me to push. The consultant came in and I was moved to theater in preparation for a c-section, my worst nightmare.

They checked my pushing power again though and got the forceps out and baby arrived. It was a horrible feeling, the head crowning! The delivery of the rest of the body was as bad as the head but then it was all over and yer man was bawling, the cheek of him! - baby, not consultant!

So now the placenta... There was a problem with it, it didn't want to move either, but with kneading and pulling it came out eventually. It was as bad as the baby! No one tells you that! I was sewn up when baby and daddy were in the recovery room and then it was off to meet the wee bugger properly and have the most delicious tea and toast ever!

Danielle's Story
I was thirty weeks pregnant and at my home in Glencree, which is about an hour's walk from town. At the time I had no car. Sometime around four a.m, I woke up with bad heart burn but managed to get back to sleep. At five thirty, I woke up again, this time with a labour pain.

At first I wasn't sure if it was labour, as I didn't think that I would be unlucky enough to have two premature babies. I had another pain at six, so I decided to get the bus to my mom's house in Bray with my partner. If I was in labour, it would be much easier to get to a hospital from there.

The bus was due at seven a.m. It is one of only three buses to come every day. I knew that if I missed it I would have no way in to Bray until eleven. So I woke up my son who was seventeen months old and started to get ready. I had another pain, followed very quickly by the urge to push. The bus stop was a twenty minute walk away. I knew I would not make it that far with such a strong urge to push.

I got my partner to ring for an ambulance and then to ring my parents. He was on one phone to my parents and on the other to the ambulance trying to give them directions to where we lived. I tried not to push but I couldn't stop myself. I gave two big pushes and my son was born.

My partner was still on the phone to the ambulance and had gone outside to try and flag them down so I had to catch my baby myself. The bag of waters broke when it came into contact with my hands. The only other person in the room was my son who had given me his favorite teddy while I was pushing. I think he wanted to make me feel better. I cleared the gunge out of his mouth and unwrapped the cord which was wound around his neck. The afterbirth came out at the same time as the baby. I didn't cut the cord as I didn't know what to do.

By then my partner was back. He gave me a blanket to wrap my son in as he was very cold and a grayish blue color I knew he was breathing as he was crying. So was I. The ambulance arrived about ten minutes after he was born. They checked me over and immediately gave him oxygen. We then went to the hospital where I was rushed straight to a ward and my son was taken straight to the intensive care unit. where he stayed for a number of weeks before eventually coming home with us.

There was a funny moment when the ambulance driver forgot to bring the after birth along to the hospital. He was supposed to bring it to be examined in order to make sure that none of it was left inside of me, but in all the commotion he forgot it. He had put it in a bag but my partner had put it in the bin so I had to get my sister and her partner to drive back to my house and collect the placenta.

Rachel's Story

I was ten days overdue with my first baby when I was brought into the hospital to be induced. I had gone private, but as luck would have it, my gynae was on holidays, so I was seen to by a lovely South African doctor who was standing in for him.

I was given an internal examination at nine am and told that my cervix was not "ripe enough" to break my waters. The doctor then proceeded to insert some prostaglandin gel and told me that he would return in six hours.

At just after three, he was back to examine me again. This time, my cervix was "unfavorable " so he inserted more gel and said that he would be back the next day.

I was SO disappointed as I was dying to meet my little one. Myself and my husband prepared ourselves for a night spent pacing the floorboards.

At around seven thirty that evening I started feeling some very sharp cramps. They were about a minute or two apart and didn't last for long but they were very painful. I called the nurse who told me that unfortunately the prostaglandin gel could cause these sorts of pains and I should take a nice long bath to try to ease the discomfort.

I did as she suggested but I found that the pains only intensified. While I was in the bath, I felt something strange, as though I had wet myself a little. Looking back now, it's pretty obvious that it must have been my waters breaking; at the time however, I figured that I was just passing the mucus plug (the show) as I had been reading about labour in so many books and I had myself convinced that this must happen before "proper" labour could commence.

I got back to the ward at around ten p.m and told the nurse that the pains were getting worse. She suggested a pethidine injection to help me sleep. I got the injection and a woozy feeling akin to that of of being incredibly drunk washed over me followed by a massive wave of nausea. My husband only just got the sick bowl to me in time before the nurse reappeared and shooed him away, telling him to go home and come back tomorrow.

I felt so lonely as I watched him walk away leaving me in pain and throwing up. This wasn't how we'd imagined things would be.

I was far too uncomfortable to sleep. Instead, I tossed and turned, biting my pillow so as not to make any noise and disturb the other women on my ward. To be honest, I probably could have let out a blood curdling scream and no one would have noticed as everyone in the room was about nine months pregnant and the chorus of snores echoing throughout the ward was reminiscent of a pneumatic drill.

At this stage the pains were coming every minute and I threw up another four times before I crept out of the ward and went down to the nurses station. It was just after midnight. I told the nurse on duty that the pethidine wasn't helping the pain at all and could she please give me something stronger. To be perfectly honest, I was a bit embarrassed at being such a nuisance. I wondered how on earth I was going to cope with labour the following day when I couldn't even manage a few piddling little prostaglandin pains!

She disappeared and returned a few minutes later with a tens machine which she gave to me to try.

Now, I had heard about these machines at my prenatal classes, but this was the first time that I had ever seen one and I really didn't know how to use it. I tried positioning the pads around me; two on my front and two on my back and then started pressing buttons on the control panel. I sat back and waited for sweet relief.

I felt nothing. No little tingle of an electric current, no pain relief – NOTHING.

I had gotten the feeling that I was annoying the nurse just a little - not that she said anything mind you - it was just the way that she was always a bit short when she spoke to me. Normally, I'd be well able to handle someone who put out those sort of vibes towards me. However, she was the one in charge of the drugs, so I kept as quiet as I could and when I felt that enough time had passed for her to believe that I had given the tens machine a good shot , I traipsed back to the Nurses station. This time, when I explained that I wasn't coping very well and didn't know how much longer I could stay quiet for, I had a few tears in my eyes and a bit of a choke in my voice.

She brought me to an examination room, attached me to a trace machine and then left me for about fifteen minutes. When she came back she examined the trace. I asked if I was in labour. She was vague and said she wasn't sure and proceeded to give me an internal examination.

All of a sudden her expression changed and she asked me when my waters had gone. It was then that I remembered the "strange feeling" in the bath and I could have kicked myself for not realizing what had happened. I was in Labour.

I could have kissed her. Despite the fact that I was in such incredible pain and getting no real break between contractions, I was finally on the way to meeting my baby . My elation though was short lived as she informed me that I was only one centimeter dilated. WHAT?!?!?!? ONE centimeter??? It was one fifteen in the morning and I had had my first pain at around half seven. At this rate it would be days before my little one made an appearance!

She told me to follow her and with that she took off at top speed down a corridor. I waddled as fast as I could through the blinding contractions, terrified that I'd lose her and a search party would have to be sent out to retrieve the silly girl who couldn't find her way across the hall. She led me to a labour room and there to my horror I met the mid-wife who was going to be looking after me.

I had met this she devil before at a prenatal appointment and while I had had very limited dealings with her, my husband and I had noticed her tending to other women and we both felt that she was a bit of a sarcastic woman who seemed to see all of the pregnant women around her as a bit of a nuisance. She was the sort of mid-wife you could imagine telling you to cop on to yourself if you dared to produce anything as new age as a birth plan.

Straight away she told me to stop fighting the pain. "Go with it" she barked, "It's bigger than you".

Well I wasn't going to argue with this bull dog of a woman, so when the next pain came, I concentrated on relaxing and just letting the pain wash over me. Lo and behold, it worked.

I was then plopped down on a birthing ball, given a cord in one hand and a gas mask in the other. The midwife was leaving the room for a moment and I was to use the cord if I needed her. As she left, she snapped at me to, "breath in the gas properly for goodness sake! Breath it in deeply!"

I quickly obeyed and promptly threw up all over the floor. I nearly died – would she give out to me when she came back? Praying that someone else would come, I took a chance and pulled the cord.

A siren sounded. The door swung open and in rushed a small army of medics with my panicked looking midwife leading the charge. Apparently, I was meant to press the little bell at the end of the cord not actually pull the cord itself.

When my husband arrived, he found me bouncing on the birthing ball, completely wrecked from hours of contractions coming one on top of the other. On his heels was the second most important man in my life - the anesthetist.

I'm not sure how fond he was of me though as the moment I was bent over his lap having the epidural administered was the moment the rest of my waters decided to let go - all over his trousers and shoes.

The next few hours were blissful compared to the ones that had gone before. I could feel the contractions but without any pain and I was even able to doze off for a while here and there!

It was during one of my little sleeps though that I began hearing whisperings about phoning the doctor and getting him to come in. I jumped awake to see a second midwife in the room. Both of them were pouring over the trace read outs. I asked what was wrong. They looked at each other and hesitated before answering.

Earlier on, I had been put on an oxytocin drip to help my labour progress and ever since then, they said, every time that I had a contraction, the baby's heart rate fell. When they turned off the drip the heart rate returned to normal. We would have to wait until the doctor came in to see what he said.

At half seven in the morning the doctor arrived to examine me. I was only four centimeters dilated. He told the midwife to turn the drip back on and to monitor the baby's heart rate. He had wanted to take a sample of blood from the baby's head to gauge a more accurate reading of how my baby was coping with the labour but the baby was too high up and I wasn't dilated enough. He said that he would be back shortly to see how things were going but I knew that he wasn't happy with how slowly the labour was progressing.

He left the room and almost straight away the baby's heart rate fell again. The midwives were changing shift and a lovely young girl sat down beside me. She was sweet and all, but suddenly, now that things were getting scary, I wanted my old battle-ax back.

The doctor returned and examined me again. I was still only four centimeters gone. He told me that he would have to section me. He was so nice and asked me if I was disappointed with that. I was, but I never said so. Instead I told him that I just wanted what was best for the baby.

People appeared from nowhere. One nurse started shaving me and inserted a catheter while another nurse started to attach pads all over my chest. Another lovely anesthetist arrived and started topping up my epidural. As I was being wheeled down the corridor he was sprinkling water all over me and asking me if I could feel it. When I said no, he declared me ready to go.

We arrived at the operating theater and I was surprised to see so many people there, everyone except my darling husband who had been taken away to be sterilized. I was nervous and threw up yet again. The doctor arrived and as he started to cut me open my husband appeared. I just clung tight to his hand.

The first cut felt like someone was unzipping me and the tugging that followed was just a tad uncomfortable – the sort of sensation that almost hurts but doesn't quite. And then I heard a little baby croaky sound. "What is it?" I shouted. The doctor told me to wait a moment as he said that baby was in a tangle. The cord was wrapped around the top of his head and twice around his neck and then my beautiful baby boy was dangled in front of me just long enough to ascertain that he was indeed, a beautiful, healthy, baby boy.

They took him into a room at the back of the theater to clean him up and weigh him and that's when I heard him let out a scream so loud that I actually jumped. I had no idea babies could scream like that. Even throughout the drama of the whole delivery, I remember hoping that this yell was a once off sort of shout. Alas, it wasn't, as I discovered over the next few weeks – mainly at two in the morning.

My husband was called to see him and minutes later he arrived back and held our son against my cheek. I couldn't get over how soft he was. Suddenly, the relief that it was all over and the knowledge that we were all safe and sound hit me like a thunderbolt. If I am to be completely honest, it was the feeling of relief that I remember far more than any feelings of love or bonding which at the time was very disappointing.

Of course the bonding and unconditional love came along shortly, but I wondered for a long time afterwards if things would have been different had I had a natural birth without complications. Would I have been lucky enough to have experienced that overwhelming joy at the moment of my son's birth? It is something I will never know so I try not to think about it any more.

Instead, I focus on the positive. Our wonderful, healthy little boy who at nearly two years old is the light of my husband's life and mine.

Kim's Story
When I was pregnant on my son, I was twenty years old and knew nothing about giving birth or pain relief. I just listened to what everybody else had to say. On the morning of my due date, I awoke with pains in my tummy and back. I rang the hospital and was told to take two tablets which I did and then drifted back to sleep until noon. I showered, dressed, put on my make up and went out for the day with my partner, who later became my husband.

After a walk and two lemonades at the pub, we went for dinner. Throughout the afternoon, the pains returned, only stronger. As we were living with my parents at the time we went back to the house and I explained to my mother how I was feeling. She told me to get my stuff and go into the hospital. We got there at eleven and I was brought up to the labour ward and told to walk for an hour. At half past twelve they broke my waters but they came out green with meconium.

As I was so young and this was my first baby, I had no idea what this meant. I went from one to ten centimeters in fifteen minutes and started pushing at three in the morning. My beautiful baby boy was born at three twenty two a.m. We barely got to look at him before he was whisked away to the special care unit.

He was there for two days and to be honest, it took a couple of weeks for me to fully bond with him. The birth also left me with a number of stitches which were very sore so it took a while to get over it!

Three and a half years later though, we decided we would like another baby. We had gotten so much joy from our son that we were looking forward to doing it again. Secretly though, I was terrified of having another frightening birth.

I was pregnant within the month and we were over the moon. Our daughter was due the twenty ninth of January and I sailed through the pregnancy. She was eleven days overdue when I started getting mild pains. At ten that night I had a show and by eleven o'clock the pains were four minutes apart. Again I was brought up to delivery and again I was told to walk for an hour which we did with our fantastic midwife. I was offered an epidural but refused it as the pain wasn't really that bad. I went back to the ward where my waters broke , I was soooooo happy to see that this time, they were clear!

75

At 3:50 that morning, after three good pushes, my baby girl was born. They handed her to us immediately and we bonded straightaway. It was the most amazing feeling ever.

The reason I wanted to tell my story is because you hear a lot of horror stories about labour. Okay, so my first time was bad but my second time was perfect! Don't be put off by other people's stories. Every birth is different. I had two very different labors and now I have two very beautiful, amazing darlings that I love with all my heart. I would do it all again, good labour or bad, because when it's all over and done, the reward is the most wonderful gift ever.

Jennifer's Stories
First Pregnancy: I woke up on the morning of my due date at about 4:30am with bad period type pains in my back. I got up and went into the bathroom for a piddle. I came back into the room and woke my husband, saying I wasn't really sure but that this could be it!!!

He got himself up and we went downstairs to ring the hospital and make a cup of tea. I talked to the nurse on the phone and she said that as I wasn't having regular contractions approximately five minutes apart, that I had a while to go yet and to try and have a shower or bath to relax.

I finished my cup of tea and went upstairs to have a shower. By the time I got into the bathroom I was crippled with contractions coming quick and strong. I Told my husband that I thought we had better leave for the hospital and shuffled away down the stairs with some help.

I was bundled into the car and we got to the hospital at about 7:00am. I was brought into a room and onto a bed. A midwife broke my waters. The pains were very strong and I had really strong urges to push. I told the midwife and she said that I wasn't to push as it was too early. She then checked me and realized I was more dilated than they though - think I was about 6 cm then - and they moved me into the delivery suite.

I was given gas and air (wonderful stuff :-))) and got through the contractions. Then came the pushing part which felt like a whole lot of work and nothing happening. Eventually Baby popped out at 8.15am.....a beautiful baby girl weighting 7lb 14oz. I needed a couple of stitches below and then got some swelling so they needed to undo stitches and then redo them... this was the worst part of the whole thing - I needed the gas and air for that...

Second Pregnancy: I woke up at 4:45am five days before my due date with those familiar period type pains in my back. I woke up my husband and he drove around to his mothers house to bring her back to mind our first baby. I got towels for the car seat in case my waters broke and downstairs into the sitting room.

My husband arrived back with my Mother in law and he ran upstairs to grab bags. My MIL timed my contractions and they were coming at two minute intervals. I Didn't really feel that bad but still wanted to get to the hospital asap as my first pregnancy was quick enough. We hopped in the car and half way there my waters broke. The contractions were really strong and painful and I was feeling that need to push.

When we got to the hospital, my husband got a wheelchair and I was taken up to the delivery suite where the midwife asked if I could give a urine sample... I just laughed and explained I couldn't even stand up. I was helped onto a bed and the midwife checked and stated that I was fully dilated and that next time I felt the urge to push to do so.

I couldn't believe it. I didn't even get the gas and air!!! twenty minutes of pushing and my son was born at 6.08am weighting in at 8lbs. I didn't need stitches thank God and an hour after he was born I was up and showering. Felt great.

On my third pregnancy, I had a watery bleed at thirty five weeks while out to dinner for our sixth wedding anniversary. We went straight into the hospital thinking that perhaps my waters had broke. When we got to the hospital I was examined and checked but they couldn't tell whether my waters had broken or not because of the blood.

They explained that I would get two steroid injections, one then and another one in twelve hours. This was to help the baby's lung development as if I did go into labour they wouldn't stop me at this stage but wanted to ensure that the baby's lungs would be developed enough. They would keep me in for the weekend and monitor the bleeding as they couldn't let me out until twenty four hours after the bleeding had stopped. I got the second steroid injection on the Saturday morning.

They explained that they needed to do an ultrasound on the Monday as they were unsure of what was causing the bleeding. I wasn't too pleased about being in hospital all weekend but what can you do? I was told that I would probably be let out after the ultrasound, so I could live with that.

Monday arrived and I went down to get my scan. I was completely devastated when she told me that I had Placenta Praevia Grade four, which meant that the placenta had fallen down and completely covered the cervix. Because of the stage I was at and the severity of my condition, I would have to have a section and would need to stay in hospital until full term. I burst into tears there and then. I couldn't believe it. I didn't know which was worse; the thought of the operation or being in hospital for the next four weeks.

When I talked to the doctor she explained that they needed to keep me in in case I had a bleed and that this was considered a high risk pregnancy as another bleed could leave me with massive blood loss and the high possibility of needing a blood transfusion. Needless to say, I was terrified as I had had it so easy with my first two births and just expected this to be the same.

The following forty eight hours, I just cried on and off worrying about who was going to look after my other two children. I didn't want my husband to use all his holidays before the baby was born, especially as having a section takes so much longer to recover from. I worried about not being there for them.

I had passed a week living in hospital when I got the date for my section. I would be just over thirty seven weeks. I was excited knowing that would be when the baby would arrive but I was definitely not looking forward to the operation.

The day arrived. I got myself showered and shaved, donned my operation gown and my lovely anti embolism socks and settled down to read. Then lo and behold, while reading and trying not to think about the upcoming op, I had a bleed.

It was quite a heavy one so the doctors were informed and they got ready to section me. Thankfully, it wasn't classed as an emergency section as I was all prepped and ready to go. I rang my husband and he arrived shortly thereafter.

As I was wheeled into the operating room I was suddenly hit with the realization that I was about to have major surgery. I was terrified and desperately trying to stay calm. Everyone was very nice and introducing themselves as they went about their business. I had about five needles in my arm and hand and what felt like three injections into my spine. These didn't hurt but were very uncomfortable and completely bizarre sensations.

I was feeling very queasy and started to panic a bit. I told them I was feeling this way and they gave me something to stop the queasiness. I felt a lot better but the whole sensation was just extremely unnatural to me. I could feel several people touching me down below but no pain. They started to cut me. I could feel it, but again there was no pain.

My husband was brought in. He could see them doing it all and later said it was very weird talking to me and seeing people cutting me open with blood everywhere at the same time. I had a screen and so couldn't see anything thank God!

I could feel pulling and tugging as they took my baby out. It was a boy, but he made no sound so they whipped him off to the other side of the room. We were delighted and surprised as I really thought it was going to be a girl. There was still no sound though.

I looked over at them and could see three people around him and a little grey hand not moving. It was too long and I started to panic. Still no sound. I started to cry, thinking that he didn't make it. It really was a very long time.

Then, thankfully, we heard an almighty scream. It was the most terrifying time of my life. He had gone into shock and his heart rate had dropped dramatically. He was placed on my chest and I felt so relieved. He was seven pounds, seven ounces. My husband then got a good proper hold of him. They explained that he was very pale and they wanted to place him in an incubator for a little bit first.

My husband and baby Adam were taken out of the room by the midwife as I was being closed up and stitched. I was then taken to another room where I waited to be checked. Baby Adam was in the room too but they said that his blood sugar levels were quite low and they felt that he needed to be fed a bottle to get his sugars up and would I be okay with this as I had wanted to breast feed. Obviously I said whatever is best for him.

I eventually got down to the ward where I got to see and spend some time with Adam and my husband. I was relieved it was all over but was not looking forward to the recovery as I couldn't move my legs at this stage. The following twenty four hours were painfully uncomfortable and just plain strange sensation wise.

They offered to take Adam away and bring him back for feeds so that I wouldn't have to change nappies and such. I didn't want to though. I said that I would do it myself but if I found it too difficult I would buzz them and let them know. I just didn't want him taken away again...

With my other two, they stayed with me from the moment they were born so I just wanted him there. I coped okay that night and each day got better and better. I got out of the hospital four days later and was feeling tender but better than I expected. Every day I get better and better but it is definitely a long and slow process compared to natural birth (for me anyway)

Mary's Story
I was one day overdue when I developed cramps mid-morning. I started to remember what my first labour was like. On my frequent trips to the bathroom, I had my three year old asking, "Have you a sore tummy Mama? Have you a sore bum?"

I didn't appreciate it at the time, but it was a good distraction. I also had to wash some dishes with him while wondering how long should I leave it before I called my partner, Noel.
I rang Noel at quarter past noon and he arrived just before one pm. As the bags were already packed, I only had to bring a bag of toys, put an old duvet cover on the back seat to go under me and put on my TENS machine. Once we were in the car, I rang the hospital to say I was on my way with twenty minutes between contractions and the staff member that answered said, "thats grand, you've loads of time".

Noel's sister was minding our son, Leon, so we had to drive to Lismore first to drop him off and by then my times had changed to fifteen minutes between contractions. At this point it was really uncomfortable sitting down, so I turned around to kneel on the back seat, with my right hand on the car seat and my left hand on the head-rest for support. I started to get really thirsty and had to stop at a garage to buy a bottle of water. I was get-

ting more painful cramps every ten minutes and at five minutes
to three, my waters broke.

I became aware of some movement in my vagina shortly after
this and when I put my hand down, I could feel the soft fuzzy
hair on my baby's head. I told Noel to stop driving and phone
999. By the time he had finished giving details of our car -
a Toyota Corolla - and location - a country back road near
Rathcormac, Co. Cork - the baby's head was after sliding out.

It was a wonderful feeling being aware of the baby turning sideways in the birth canal and shortly after, my girl was born at
five minutes past three. I never had the urge to push that I hear
other women have and she pretty much delivered herself.

Ten minutes after her birth, the guards arrived to check on us as
is standard response to a 999 call. I wasn't sure how long more
the ambulance would take, so I gave her her very first breastfeed
in the back seat of the car, just seconds after the placenta volun-
tarily came out itself.

My daughter Esme was about twenty five minutes old when
the ambulance arrived and they were surprised to see that the
birth was over. One of the staff cut the cord and took us to the
hospital for a check up. I gave her a second feed in the ambulance, just in case things got hectic in the hospital and I missed
a chance to do it later.

Other then needing stitches for a few small tears, we were
both declared well and healthy. I wanted to go home on day
two, but I stayed in hospital for a few days extra so we could
register her birth in the hospital registry office before we left.
Unfortunately, our stay was for naught as because Esme wasn't
born in the hospital, we could not register her birth there and
would instead have to go to the nearest office to the location
of her birth!

Real Mams Talk About:
Birth

Don't be surprised if you feel a bit disconnected from things after the birth. It took a day or so for everything to sink in with me, I felt like I was on autopilot some of the time. I also wish I had been firmer about people coming to the hospital without prior notice, some visitors seemed to think it was acceptable to wake me up if I was asleep when they arrived unannounced.

Lara, 28, Meath

I suppose to try and be as fit as possible for the birth. It's hard work and if you're getting an epidural, it can end up being a long process.

Jane, 32, Dublin

Listen to no-one. Your experience will be so different... make it your own and relax... you know best. Don't be told what to do by anyone.

Ciara, 33, Dublin

Have a birth plan but don't expect to stick to it word for word. I was quite happy to do whatever the midwives and my consultant suggested as I found them to be fantastic and very understanding. One thing I really advise is to take an hour or two to yourselves as a new family before any visitors arrive no matter how desperate the doting grandparents, aunts and uncles are to see the new arrival. We really enjoyed that time together.

Ingrid, 29, Cavan

At the time you think it is the worst thing in the world but you do actually forget what the pain felt like and once you have that tiny baby in your arms it makes it all worthwhile.

Leanne, 26, Donegal

You can do it. Just keep thinking through each contraction that it's one more push towards meeting your baby. I had a little sock in my hand the whole time to remind me of this. The high you experience after is like no other.

Fiona, 28, Kildare

Chapter Five

BIRTH STORIES II: STAYING HOME

"When I think of giving birth, the only word that comes to me is "Primal." I know it's the most natural thing to happen, but I felt a power inside me that, whenever I find life getting too difficult for me, I bring back that primal feeling and know that if I can give birth with no pain relief or surgery/stitches, then I can do anything. I don't think I was scared but I was stubborn. When I got into a position, I wouldn't move as I knew I was safe. When my son was born, I loved how the midwife put him in my arms without telling me whether he was a boy or girl, she left that for me to discover. He held my finger, opened his eyes and looked up at me and all that pain was forgotten."

Mandy, 24, Cork

I never thought I'd be on the computer whilst in labour, but, TA DAAAH! Here I am! After several small incidents in the night where I worried that I'd completely lost control of my bladder, I finally twigged and realized that my waters had broken and that the pains I was feeling were not indigestion from the waaaayyyy over priced Madras curry I'd eaten for supper (Rice not included in price...wtf?!?!?) but were indeed the start of labour. Which is where I am now... hanging out in my kitchen, contracting away whilst the new baby moves ever closer to being born.

Happy Birthday Baby! See you soon:)

Sheena's Story

It is a long and convoluted journey that led me from hospital to home birth. But in a nutshell, it was the fact that my first baby was born by section that led me ultimately to choose a home birth for my third baby.

I have never been given a medical reason for my first baby being born by section. I have received copies of my hospital notes which don't give one either. The approach taken by my consultant (I was a private patient) runs counter to my understanding of best practice (to put it mildly).

At full-term, my waters broke but I had no contractions. My consultant put me on an oxytocin drip immediately, despite having told me twelve hours earlier that my cervix was in no way favorable

From the outset, he appeared to have neither interest nor faith in my ability to give birth. It seemed he just wanted to get things finished so he could go home. At no time was I or my baby in distress. Fifteen hours after my waters went I was given two hours, "to make considerable progress" or he would carry out a section.

Not surprisingly I didn't and he did. It was a sad and frightening introduction to motherhood, an experience that I never wanted to repeat. I was thirty three years old, highly educated, extremely fit and healthy. I came from a family where drug-free, natural births were the norm. I'd had a problem free pregnancy and had every expectation that the birth would be the same. Almost nine years later, I am still angry about how I was treated and that I allowed it.

On my second pregnancy, I was not naive enough to believe that I could or should trust the system to instinctively work with me. I was better informed about the maternity system and ready to take greater responsibility for my care.

I switched hospitals and the form of care I opted for. I wanted every possible chance to give birth to my baby vaginally. The hospital I chose to go to had a lower section rate than the hospital where my first baby was born and it had a good vbac rate. I chose semi-private care to avoid having a consultant hanging over me on the day. I wanted midwife led care and my first preference would have been the Community Midwives but I was excluded from the scheme because of my previous section. Even a letter to the Master couldn't change that, despite the fact that I was happy to have my baby in hospital.

I saw a fantastic consultant for my appointments . He was hugely supportive and on the day turned out to be instrumental in taking the decision to wait for my body to go into labour itself. I am eternally grateful to him for that.

My second labour started as my first had, with my waters breaking but no contractions. This time however, I was allowed to wait to go into labour, though that wait had to be in hospital. Seventy-three hours after my waters broke I gave birth to my second son. Despite the fact that this was still a highly medicalized birth – I'd had two shots of pethidine, gas and air, oxytocin, an epidural and an episiotomy - I was overjoyed.

That said, we found the whole experience very stressful. The hospital felt so foreign to me. The monitor, aka "the machine that went beep," unnerved me. The need to perform to a schedule that just didn't fit with my body's, put me on edge.

Before I was even pregnant with baby number three I was pretty sure that this time, I wanted to go the home birth route. I wanted to give birth without having to do it against the clock. None of the hospitals and associated consultant led care would give me that option and I was still excluded from the community midwife led schemes.

As soon as I got my positive test result I was on the phone to my midwife of choice, a formidable woman with a wealth of experience who handily lives only a few minutes away. Both my husband and I were very comfortable with her down to earth, matter-of-fact, straight-talking approach. The decision was made.

From the outset my c-section was a non-issue, and my age (I was just about to turn 41) was never even mentioned. As far as my midwife was concerned, I was fit and healthy, I had a history of problem free, textbook pregnancies, my scar had been "tested" successfully and I was a good candidate for a home birth. The fact that she was happy made me happy. I trusted her experience and she trusted my body. What a novelty!

As my estimated due date approached, I was irritated at still being pregnant and apprehensive about how much longer I'd have to wait. This baby felt and looked big. I was tired of waddling and eager to meet my new baby who I was convinced was a third boy. My intuition had been reliable both previous times so why not this time?

Two days before my due date was a beautiful day in what had been a very mixed summer. I spent it hanging out with the boys and my dad. A friend had phoned to tell me that she was as cranky as a wasp in the days before her son was born. I laughed, wishing that that could explain my bad temper but I didn't really take it to heart. Little did I know!

My dad had just left the house when my waters went at about four pm. As both of my previous labors had started that way but with no contractions I didn't expect much to happen. But this time, contractions started within a very short time. My midwife dropped in at about four thirty, checked the baby's heartbeat and said to call if anything started. When my husband, Alan, arrived home at five, he could tell when I was having contractions, even though I was doing my best to ignore them as I made dinner for the boys.

Even though labour on my second son, Daniel, had stopped and started over a period of days, we decided at about six thirty that Alan should take the boys to his parents, so we must have had some sense of things going somewhere.

When the midwife texted again at seven thirty to see if there had been any change, I texted back that pains had started and were now four to five minutes apart. When my midwife got my text, she phoned me. I had a contraction while she was on the phone and she said she'd be right over. I was a bit surprised, so I was obviously still in denial. She arrived just as Alan got back from dropping off the boys. She asked permission and then gave me an internal exam (the only one she did). I was two centimeters dilated and my cervix was soft. Everything was looking good.

I labored in the kitchen as the table was just the right height for leaning on. The back doors were thrown open and I spent some time in the doorway looking out on the summer evening. I couldn't sit down and found myself getting tired and shaky in my legs as things went on. I felt I should eat something to keep my energy up but I threw up after a couple of bites of toast so that was the end of that.

At around nine pm, I got into the birthing pool. The relief between contractions was extraordinary. Absolutely blissful! I felt I got some rest even though things moved on and as I reached the pushing stage nothing was really registering except a realization that I'd never done this before and had no idea what it was that I was "supposed" to be doing. I pointed this out to my midwife several times but she patiently explained that I didn't need to 'know' anything. I wasn't convinced!

I was increasingly tired and annoyed with this baby who just didn't seem to be interested in coming out (though my midwife later pointed out, the slow exit was why I only had an unstitchworthy tear when my 9lb3oz baby appeared at 11:18 that night!) The sensations as the baby descended were very strange: I felt like there was a giant walnut moving about inside me, not a smooth skulled baby.

I spent practically the whole time on all fours draped over the edge of the pool. I tried turning over briefly but hated the feeling of lying back. Apparently time was passing, though I'd no sense of it. Eventually a head appeared followed a couple of pushes later by the slither of a body. I greeted my beautiful baby 'boy' and only a few minutes later when the midwife asked what we'd had did Alan move the cord to show me how wrong I was. We had a daughter and the boys had a much wanted sister. She latched on in the pool and at some point the cord was cut. I got out of the pool after a little and Alan held Beth (as we later named her) while I delivered the placenta, showered and was tucked up in bed.

After the midwife had left, Alan, Beth and I shared some precious 'us time' together before falling asleep. When the boys came home the next day, they greeted their sister with total delight and no sense of the hiatus that Sam had experienced with my disappearance into hospital to have Daniel and my reappearance five days later with a baby in tow.

I can't begin to describe what the experience was to me. Having had a birth by c-section, and a vbac (vaginal birth after cesarean) complete with continuous monitoring, oxytocin, pethidine, gas and air, an epidural, and episiotomy, I had no 'reason' to believe that I could give birth naturally, except for a deep-seated belief that I could, given the right support and the right environment. I felt a need to reclaim my body and its capabilities from those that had undermined the belief that I had grown up with. It was tough briefly but it was an extraordinary experience. I'd never felt the actual birthing before and found the sensations very strange and not at all what I'd expected.

It was so lovely to be home. I felt safe throughout. I never had to make a conscious decision that I was in labour, I just was. One thing led to another, and another, and then my baby was there. I never felt at risk. I never felt the jolts of stress that punctuated my hospital experiences where monitors beeped and blipped throughout labour.

Home was everything I'd hoped, everything I knew it to be. I am still bowled over by what a contrast it has been to previous experiences and I feel genuinely blessed in having had the experience. I also feel more than a little sad that such an experience will not be available to other mums with a section in their past but that's another day's work.

I am, and will remain, eternally grateful to my fabulous midwife for walking the path she does and for the opportunity that she gave to me.

Samantha's Story

Not long after I realized I was pregnant for the second time, I spent many sleepless nights getting excited about the thought of having this baby at home. I wanted to do it with our first baby, Megan, but we were staying at my parents half renovated house and it just didn't seem like the right place.

I decided to invite all the females in my family to the birth; in fact this was a big factor in wanting a home birth. You can only have one person with you at a hospital birth and that was obviously going to be my husband, Ben. I read a lot about home birth and realized that in years past, most women would've seen a birth long before they experienced it themselves. I thought it might be nice for some of the girls in the family to have that experience. Also, I am very much in favor of women giving birth with no intervention - or as little as possible - and that, of course, is more likely to happen in the peace of your own home.

The first thing I had to do was find a midwife who would be willing to attend me at my own home. Not such an easy task when you consider that there just aren't all that many independent midwives in Ireland and that most of them live in big cities. The home birth website gave me a couple of names and phone numbers. The midwife I made contact with was on holiday in Italy at the time but returned my call and promised to come see me when she came home. I sent her a letter with some of my maternity history so she could read through it when she returned. At the beginning of August she came to visit and agreed to take me on.

By the end of August, my midwife had established monthly visits and all the organizing was underway. She recommended one trip to book in at the hospital and have blood tests and a scan done, which I did. It's better to have a file open at the hospital in case of emergency.

While waiting for my scan and my bloods, I had a great read through all the notes taken on my last pregnancy and birth. I also managed to have an argument with the consultant who was immediately negative about home birth. My family doctor had told me not to be "too disappointed," when I told him my plans. Neither reaction surprised me; they were both men and both in the medical profession with its highly sterilized, medicalized, women-can't-do-it-alone attitude to birth.

But I'm sure they meant well.

It was lovely having my midwife come to my home for her regular visits and to completely avoid Doctor's waiting rooms and Maternity clinics for all those months. To be seen in your own home by one person with the experience of delivering thousands of babies was wonderful.

As the big day drew nearer, I was convinced that I would go early or at least on time. For about a month I was constantly having strong Braxton-Hicks contractions. Everyone said that was the way it often is in a second pregnancy. I had a lot of pressure on my pelvis so it felt like I was constantly running for the bathroom. Sleeping was getting harder and harder. Then, in the week I was due, I came down with whatever illness was doing its rounds.

After a particularly bad night of hardly sleeping and not being able to breathe, when I was five days overdue, I was worried that I was so ill that there was no way I could cope with labour. I didn't want to take antibiotics this close to breastfeeding, so instead, I booked in with an acupuncturist who was also a mid-wife. That relieved things a bit and the next day I had an ap-pointment at the chiropractor who I was by now paying weekly visits to. I didn't want my pelvis misaligned for the important task of birthing! The treatments made me feel a little better and like I'd done all I could to improve the situation. The midwife assured me on Tuesday that if I did go into labour that night all my symptoms would disappear anyway because the adrenalin would kick in. This was comforting.

Wednesday morning, the 31st of January 2008 dawned and I was weepy and miserable. Family members came to take Megan out for the day. I wasn't coping too well. By mid morning, I felt that I was getting light contractions and didn't dare to hope. At lunch time I'd asked my Mom to come around so we could take a walk. I texted the midwife and said 'something was happen-ing...' light contractions and a big bowel clear out and clearly the weepiness meant hormones! But I still didn't want to get too excited until things were more obvious. I let both my sisters-in-law know that maybe they'd be seeing a birth tonight!

After a walk and some tidying around the house, the contrac-tions were still coming; a few were a little stronger. We took the travel cot down to my brother's house in case Megan had to stay there the night. Whilst there, I felt a pop and a strong contraction and when I went to the bathroom, had a show. Then the contractions got really strong and started coming closer together so we called the midwife who said she was on her way. Then I got a bit panicky and asked Mom to ring Ben and request him to come home immediately.

We went back to my house. I thought some hoovering would take my mind off it all. I couldn't keep that up for long though. The contractions were getting too strong. My midwife called to see how I was doing and when she heard how strong and close the contractions were, advised me to get on all fours with my bum in the air to take pressure off the cervix. This helped. I was sending her a text message with directions as to how to get to our house quickly because she was stuck in traffic. My Dad had popped in and thought it was quite amusing to see me down behind the kitchen table on all fours, moaning and texting. Ben came in at some point and I started ordering him and Mom around so that things could be made ready.

I'm sure it was around 5:00pm that things got very intense. Mom was getting everything prepared; Judah had dropped the screen off and I was moaning quietly but forgetting to breathe over the pains. She reminded me to and this helped. In between contractions I was worried about Megan having her dinner which was just cooked. Then I wanted Ben to help me get cleaned up so we headed up to the bathroom which was not easy! I got into the bath and was really having strong contractions with not much time in between to recover. I told Ben that I felt I was going to have a bowel movement and then it dawned on us that it was actually the urge to push! Ben said he could see a bulge in my back as the baby started to move down the birth canal.

I just about got dried and put on my birth shirt and made it back downstairs. Then I just started to roll about on the 'space hopper' which Mom had bought in place of a birth ball. My brother had kindly blown it up half an hour before. I was crying a little to myself as the contractions got really strong. Alison arrived at some point but no midwife and no Adriana. I wasn't worried about the midwife not being there. I had confidence that Ben and Mom could help me deliver and I was too focused on myself and the pain to care much about anything anyway. I heard Mom make some phone calls telling Adriana to get home from shopping or she was going to miss the birth and then a relived note to her voice as she spoke to the midwife who said she was just getting close to town.

The last half hour of the birth gets blurry. I remember having very strong urges to push but holding back a little too. In between contractions I was totally lucid and rested for a few seconds. The midwife asked Ben for a torch. He said he didn't have one and I reminded him that he did in the van. When he got it, the midwife put it on and said it was too bright. I agreed. I'd had all the curtains closed and just some candles burning and that was all the light I wanted. It made me feel cocooned and not so exposed.

When the contractions got really intense, Mom got down on the floor in front of me and held my hand and breathed with me. Then Ben got down too. In the end, for all the contractions - especially the pushing ones - I held onto an arm of each of them and gripped them as I moved forward and into the contraction. It really helped. I couldn't have done it without them. I labored on all fours, all the time leaning on the ball and the midwife checking the progress and then putting the tail of my shirt back down again. Adriana and Alison were standing quietly behind me watching it all unfold.

At the start of the pushing when the midwife arrived, she said, 'you're doing really well... take your time. You're stretching nicely.' And then when a little more time had passed, she said a couple more pushes and your baby will be out. But no! A couple more pushes and I kept feeling the baby slide back in!

About ten pushes later (it had to have been that many!) and finally my baby slipped out and was caught by our midwife, all in one gigantic, burning push and contraction!

I sat back on my haunches and the midwife passed my brand new, slippery, baby crying lustily under my legs to me. My Mom immediately wanted to know what we had and I moved the umbilical cord to discover that we had another beautiful daughter. Then I remembered Adriana and Alison behind me and told them to come around and see. Mom and Ben had kinda missed the moment of birth by being in front of me helping me through the pushing but it all happens so fast anyway, that you could blink and miss it!

I sat there on my living room floor, euphoric. I'd done it again! Everyone else was crying, Mom, Ben, Adriana and Alison. My tears came later when Megan met her new sister.

The midwife said that the placenta might take up to an hour to deliver. I sat back on some pillows to cushion my sore rear end but then felt some more contractions so it was time to cut the cord suddenly. Ben didn't enjoy the job anymore the second time around but he did it and then someone took the baby; I suppose it was Ben. I went to the bathroom to deliver the placenta within minutes of delivering Hayley.

Once I was cosy in my bed, the midwife gave the girls, Ben and Mom an anatomy lesson on the placenta. She pronounced it very healthy, showed them the maternal side and the side the baby was cocooned in, along with the sack she stayed safely in for her nine months residence in my womb. It was truly amazing to look at. Ben showed me the next day before burying it in our back garden!

Meg had been right all along that I was carrying a girl. Everyone else prophesied a boy! After a bit, everyone was shooed out of the bedroom and Megan was sent off with her present, a baby doll. Then the midwife weighed, checked and dressed Hayley. She was a surprising 8lb 9ozs and 51cm long!

It took awhile to settle down from the high we were on. Ben and I didn't sleep until well after midnight. Megan went to her own bed, not even having to spend one night away from home.

And now Hayley is six days old, feeding like her life depends on it, which it does! She's quite a contended little lady. She already recognizes a breast coming toward her and likes to look at shadows. Like all newborns, she smells good enough to eat and her breath is like perfume when she's just had her milk. It sounds like she's crying for some now so I'd better go feed my second daughter.

B's Story
I had my first child in hospital at thirty four weeks, so the possibility of a home birth had not really crossed my mind when I was expecting number two. However, baby had other plans and we simply did not make it to the hospital.

By the time the ambulance arrived, they refused to take me anywhere without a doctor present, so they called for one but she wasn't any help either. Supposed to do nothing but accompany me to the hospital which was twenty minutes away and fully aware why she was being called out in the first place, she stood in front of me and called out, " What am I going to do with you?" Not the thing you want to hear when you're in labour!

Anyway, one of the guys spotted the card of a midwife I had done my antenatal classes with next to my phone and asked me did I think she might come if he gave her a call? Said and done, she was there within thirty minutes and she was eight months pregnant herself at the time!

Well, to cut a long story short, son number two was born at 2:52 am. Apart from the surprise at not making it to the hospital and the useless doctor, it was a lovely experience once the midwife had arrived. From then on, I always said that should I have any more children I'd like to have them at home.

When I got pregnant again in 2004 we were living in Dublin and just outside the area where a home birth would have been available for me. However, we moved to Cork when I was around twenty weeks pregnant. Getting set up with an independent midwife under the home birth scheme in Cork was no problem at all. I had a lovely and quite fast delivery in January 2005 and then another lovely birth (even faster) with the same midwife in Feb 2006.

Having moved yet again, I am planning to have another home birth in December with another midwife, working under the home birth scheme in Cork and am very much looking forward to it.

Diane's Story

It was fantastic! Finally, I had the experience I was longing for since my first pregnancy. It was my third baby, but my first home birth. The midwife came immediately when I rang her saying that the baby was coming that night. I was two or three cm dilated when she arrived, and she let me do whatever I wanted.

I listened to my hypno birthing cd and sat on the birthing ball for a while. When my second daughter woke up at 2:00 am, I breastfed her while still sitting on the ball and having very manageable cramps.

After that, my parents took her downstairs and my husband massaged my back with clary sage oil during each contraction. They became stronger and more frequent, but still very manageable as I used a deep breathing technique I had learned from a pregnancy yoga dvd. All the time, I was leaking water every so often.

Then I felt a lot of pressure and I lay down on my left side again (I had been sitting on the edge of the bed during the last half hour) and with my husband behind me, I breathed through the next few contractions as my baby moved down the birth canal. She was two pounds bigger than my first and second, so I was a bit overwhelmed. The other two had easily slipped down and this wasn't so easy... But then the head was there. It was born during one contraction in which the midwife got me to blow and push alternately.

The next contraction I pushed the shoulders out and the rest of her body just slipped out along with a big gush of waters. It was so beautiful and empowering, and the midwife was there for me whenever I needed her but was very calm and kept in the background. My husband went downstairs to get my second daughter so she could see her baby sister. The baby latched on to my breast very easily and she knew what to do right away. She had three good feeds while we waited for the placenta to be born.

The next morning my first daughter, who slept through it all, got to see her new baby sister as well. It was a wonderful, natural, birth. The midwife only used homeopathic remedies when needed. There were no interventions and she didn't check for dilation after the first time either, but trusted my body instead. I found that excellent. Of course if the labour had lasted longer she would have had to check every four hours, but from the time I had my second daughter on the breast to the birth was only two hours and forty minutes and the contractions only really got going after that feed.

Bill's Birth

Initially, arranging a home birth wasn't easy. At just five weeks pregnant, I tried to find a midwife but each of the four midwives who cover the Dublin area was either booked up for July or planning to be away at that time. I then contacted Holles Street to see if I could join the domino scheme but was turned away as I live outside the catchment area.

Plan C was to book into Our Lady of Lourdes in Drogheda and hope that I would be allocated a place on the Midwife Led Unit. As the MLU scheme is still a randomized trial, I was told that I had a two in three chance of getting a place but that I wouldn't find out if I was successful until after my first appointment at seventeen weeks – some three months down the line. It wasn't ideal but the alternative was booking into a Dublin hospital so I decided to take my chances with Drogheda. At sixteen weeks however, fate intervened.

An independent midwife called me to say she could take me on and I breathed a sigh of relief. I liked K immediately. She was knowledgeable, kind and funny and her expertise inspired confidence. Each visit reinforced my decision to give birth at home.

Towards the end of the pregnancy, people constantly remarked that I must be dying for it to be over with. But I really wasn't. While the baby was due on July seventh, I fully expected to go at least two weeks past this date. Both my sisters and my mother had gone two weeks over on many of their births and I was confident that the baby would be born on or after July twenty first. At the time, we were extending the house and renovating our bathroom and the job wasn't due for completion until mid July so I really hoped that the baby wouldn't come on time. I was also attending a series of hypnobirthing classes and I wanted to complete these before labour began. But the best laid plans....

Following a very straightforward and enjoyable pregnancy, my labour started at one thirty in the morning on Monday, July tenth, three days past my due date. Since I work for myself, I hadn't yet managed to start my maternity leave. I had some work still due so I was working late at home on the Sunday night. When I tried to go to bed at half past one, I realized that I was too uncomfortable to lie down. This was new since I had had no trouble sleeping throughout the pregnancy. I was experiencing very mild period-like pains in my lower back at regular intervals – perhaps ten minutes apart.

I went back to the study to work and put my hypnobirthing CD on to play. This is how I spent the night, working at the desk, pausing occasionally to breathe through the discomfort of the contractions but recognizing that they weren't causing any real pain. I don't recall actively listening to the CD – rather, every forty minutes or so, I realized that it had come to an end and I would press play again. Mostly I just concentrated on getting the work finished. I still wasn't convinced that this was labour since it seemed much too manageable.

At about four a.m, I had a show and I started to think it might be happening for real. At this point, I woke Aidan. I remember distinctly that his reaction to the news that I was probably start-ing labour was, "Oh bollocks." Then he rolled over and went back to sleep. I felt reassured that he was behaving normally and not jumping around panicking. I've no time for those an-tics! I went back to the office and continued to work.

The builders were due at the house at eight that morning. At around seven, Aidan asked me if I wanted to cancel them. I told him that they should come ahead since the contractions were so mild that I could be in labour for days. It was my brother-in-law's firm that was doing the work. When they ar-rived, Aidan told Brian what was happening and he and his team focused on getting the new kitchen finished, painted and as ready as possible to give birth in.

Aidan kept asking me to ring K, but I was reluctant since I still felt that I was a long way off of established labour. At about nine thirty a.m, I called her just to let her know that something had started. She said she'd do a few visits first and see me later. She knew from the sound of my voice that I was nowhere close to needing her. After that, I phoned my mum. It was funny since I was very calm and very practically-minded. I wanted to ask her to collect a couple of items that I still hadn't gotten around to getting, like a birthing ball and other bits and pieces, but as soon as I heard her voice, I started to cry. I was obviously quite emotional just below the surface.

The morning continued with the contractions coming somewhat more frequently and gaining slightly in intensity. I still couldn't describe them as painful. I was no longer playing the CD, but just trying to get the work finished. Aidan was a terrific help, since by this time, the phone had started to ring and he fielded calls and managed to deal with lots of work queries without once mentioning to anyone that I was in labour.

At eleven thirty, I got into the shower, assuming that it would be a comfort. I stood, directing the spray onto my back but quickly found that it became uncomfortable. I got out of the shower and got dressed. I found it easier to sit upright through the contractions.

At around noon, my mum and sister arrived, and it was just lovely to see them. They stayed only a short time but it was a relaxed visit; I felt fine and the contractions still felt okay. I tried the birthing ball for a time, but found it awkward so I abandoned it.

K arrived at about half one and encouraged me to try to sleep. She did ask if I would like to be examined but I wasn't keen on the idea. While I knew I was most likely still in the latent phase, I don't think I wanted confirmation that I hadn't even started to dilate. K didn't pursue it. She attached the tens machine and put it to the lowest setting. She suggested that I play around with it but I just didn't feel inclined to interfere and it remained at that setting all day. I really can't say with any certainty whether it helped or not.

After some point, K arranged the pillows on my bed and I lay down on my side while she sat on the edge of the bed and chatted. K sent Aidan out to buy hot water bottles and she placed two of them on my back and side. They felt lovely. I think her intention was to have me fall asleep, since I had already lost a night's sleep and the birth was most likely a long way off. But I couldn't fall asleep and I found the contractions more difficult to cope with lying down. They felt intense at the peak, but they still seemed very short – no more than twenty seconds in duration and coming every four or five minutes or so.

At about five pm, I heard Brian and all the builders leaving. K asked if she could examine me and this time I agreed. I suppose I was curious. It was the first and last vaginal examination of the pregnancy and birth and was over very quickly. She announced that I was between four and five centimeters dilated. I was delighted since I still felt that the contractions weren't too bad at all. K told me that I was sufficiently dilated to get into the birthing pool and she and Aidan headed downstairs to set it up. I continued to lie on the bed for a short time but eventually felt I'd cope better standing up.

There was a pile of towels and sheets sitting on the chest of drawers which reached chest height. I found it helpful to stand and lean into the pile and bury my face in the towels at the height of a contraction.

After a while, I headed downstairs where Aidan and K were filling the pool with some difficulty since the tap/ hose connection wasn't working. I was struck by how perfect the setting was. That morning, the extension had been full of rubble and building equipment. Now it was a huge, empty box with the evening sunshine streaming through the windows. The guys had painted the walls and bonded the concrete floor. It mightn't sound like everyone's idea of a perfect birth setting but I was thrilled with it.

I wandered about a bit, watching as K and Aidan continued to fill the pool, and sending text messages to my mum and sisters. After a time, I went back upstairs in search of the pile of laundry and brought it down to the kitchen counter, leaning into the contractions once more. I didn't know it at the time, but the trips up and down the stairs were helping to move the baby down.

At this point, the contractions had begun to change. They were still manageable and I still got great relief from the gap between them, but they were more intense and coming every two or three minutes. I started to feel a sort of bulging pressure in my bum at the end of each one. I told K and she just nodded and told me that was fine. The contractions still felt no more than twenty five seconds in length. And between contractions, I felt completely normal – as though I wasn't in labour at all.

At about ten to seven, the pool was ready and I got in. I know many women describe the sensation of getting in to the pool as miraculous and while I did find it pleasant, it wasn't radically different. I sat in the pool and continued to feel those pushy, bulgy contractions. K instructed Aidan to give me a cold, wet facecloth, which he did. I hadn't looked for it, had no idea I wanted it, but it was just lovely. With each contraction, I buried my face in the icy, wet cloth.

After a while, K suggested that I feel what was happening. I put my hand down and felt the bag of waters bulging. It was a peculiar sensation! Shortly afterwards, I felt the waters break with a loud pop. At some point, K gave me some homeopathic remedies to suck but I don't recall which ones they were.

At one point, Aidan came over and put his arms around me but I pushed him away. I was concentrating hard and I had sort of retreated into myself. I didn't want the contact or the distraction although I was very glad of his presence at a distance. K asked me if I wanted some gas and air but I couldn't bear the thought of any interference or of putting a mask over my face. The contractions were gaining in intensity and coming more frequently but there was always a gap between them which made them manageable. I was pretty much silent throughout all the contractions.

K asked me if I wanted to get out of the pool to give birth. But I had no desire to move and there was no way I was leaving the pool. I felt I was going further into myself. I continued to kneel in the pool, leaning over the edge, with my face in the cloth.

A few minutes later, K knelt down beside me and told me that the baby was coming, that I should push on the next contraction. I said no and turned my head in the opposite direction. She came around to the other side and repeated it very gently. And so, on the next contraction I pushed and the baby's head was born. Somehow, I had raised my hips so that the head emerged from the water. K told me to stay raised so that the baby's head wouldn't be re-submerged. In what was only seconds, I felt the baby's body come out and heard a loud cry. It was 7:40pm.

I continued to lean over the edge of the pool for a few moments. I think I was almost afraid to turn around to look at the baby. K and Aidan coaxed me around, both refusing to tell me if it was a boy or a girl. I turned and saw it was a boy. I was surprised since I had become convinced towards the end of the pregnancy that I was carrying a girl. He looked very big and very red and very beautiful. I raised one leg and K maneuvered him under and into my arms. I sat back down in the pool and cuddled him. It was an extraordinary feeling. The chord was quite short and it stopped pulsating very soon. K clamped it, Aidan cut it and baby Bill and I were separated for the first time. K produced a baby sheepskin and wrapped him in it. Aidan held him while I stood in the pool and delivered the placenta.

Then it was out of the pool, and immediately upstairs to bed where K set about getting Bill properly latched on and feeding. K stood beside the bed, and patiently latched and re-latched the baby until he took to it. It must have taken an hour and I remember wondering, where's the lovely tea and toast that everyone talks about after birth? But the breastfeeding has worked like a charm with no problems whatsoever. In hindsight, I know that it is because of K's efforts. After the first hour, Aidan appeared with tea and bacon and eggs and we all ate sitting around the bed. The baby was weighed and we discovered that he was eight pounds exactly.

We made our calls to the family to let them know that Bill had arrived. My other sister and her husband (Brian the builder) called around briefly to meet the boy.

K stayed the first night. And I'm embarrassed to say that with the building work going on, she was forced to sleep on a dusty sofa in a rubble filled sitting room. When the baby woke during the night to feed, she came up and sat with me while I tried to get it right, gently advising and helping with the positioning.

The next morning, she ran me a bath and then took the baby while I soaked. I came back to find a beautifully made up bed with a mountain of pillows. She then bathed the boy and tucked him up beside me. She left that morning only after ensuring that I had everything I needed by my side.

I lay on the bed watching my amazing son and feeling tired but so, so happy. K continued to visit daily for ten days after the birth and weekly after that until he was six weeks old. The fabulous post-natal care was a revelation and one of the surprise bonuses of the whole experience.

Home birth has been the most rewarding experience. I had been skeptical about hypno birthing and though I never actively thought about it during the labour and birth, I'm sure that it must have played a part.

I didn't have a pain-free labour but it was wonderful nonetheless. The contractions were always manageable. I kept waiting for it to get really hard but it never did. I think the single most important factor was that I was never, ever afraid. I'm convinced that fear sabotages childbirth. Throughout the entire birth I felt confident, safe and secure, in my own home with Aidan and with K.

Real Mams Talk About:
Home birth...
I'm from the Netherlands where home birth is widely accepted and normal, but had my first two children here in Ireland, in the hospital. I wasn't very happy with the way consultants just take over and decide by their own agendas when the baby should come instead of giving a mother's body a chance to go into labour herself. I've been induced twice, the first time barely over my due date and the second time two weeks early. I found out way later that there wasn't even any real reason for it. My second child especially would have been much better off to stay where she was for another two weeks at least. She was so sleepy and jaundiced, and only started picking up health-wise after her original due date. So the main reason to go for a home birth this time is to get a more natural approach. This time I don't feel pressured to have the baby by my due date and am much more relaxed.

Diane, 27, Dublin

I benefited from the combined experience of my mum and my two older sisters; all three went through the hospital system themselves but encouraged me to explore natural or low intervention birth options. I started reading up before I even became pregnant and the more I read, in books and on-line, the more I understood that the odds of having a natural birth are stacked against you in a hospital, especially first time out. I recall reading the annual report from my local maternity hospital and discovering that only five percent of first time mothers give birth spontaneously without any form of intervention or instrumental delivery. Meanwhile, I was also reading birth accounts from home birthers and I was completely won over by their enthusiasm for delivering at home. Shortly after getting a positive pregnancy test, I attended a home birth meeting and I was hooked on the idea.

Bill's Mam

Do your research, talk to lots of different people, talk to the midwives and realize they are the experts in normal birth. Trust your body and be comfortable with what you choose.

Karen, 27, Cork

With my second child, I wanted to avoid the feelings of helplessness and inadequacy I experienced with my first birth, which was in hospital. I wanted to be allowed to labour at my own pace, in the comfort of my own home, surrounded by the people I love. I wanted my baby to delivered by someone who knew me and to whom I was more then just a number.

Lisa, 28, Cork

I have a reputation for being a bit impulsive and I think when I first started talking about having a home birth, they took it with a pinch of salt. I did have an aunt I'm very close to beg me not go through with it as she felt it was putting our safety at risk unnecessarily, but I explained that midwives are so used to the birthing process that things rarely go wrong without warning signs and that at the first sign of anything unusual, we'd be off to hospital. Once I explained that it wasn't some fanciful idea we had, that it was a well researched and logical decision, the majority of people were happy to support us. But at the end of the day, once my hubby was behind me, I wasn't asking for anyone's permission!

Pamela, 28, South Tipperary

We were selective in who we told. I'm not an evangelist looking to convert others. I didn't see why I should have to defend our decision. I didn't want to worry others. And I didn't want others to antagonize us. We had researched our decision. We knew that others hadn't.

Sheena, Dublin

My GP told me that something WOULD happen during my pregnancy and I WOULD end up in hospital. No ifs, ands or buts about it. My mother went as far as PAYING a private consultant and making an appointment for me. The few people that didn't think I was making a big mistake told me I'd regret it when I needed pain killers. As for my partner, he was worried at first, but he also thought that being together at home would be a much nicer experience, and he was definitely keen on being able to stay with me and the baby instead of having to spend the first night at home alone. Once we realized how safe it was, he was right behind me.

For anyone thinking about home birth, I'd recommend that you get your hands on the booklet published by the Southern Health Board, entitled, "Domiciliary Midwifery Pilot Project for Cork City & County - Evaluation of the Southern Health Board Home Birth Pilot Project." Read it, and show the statistics to worried family and friends. It's based in Cork, so there is no room for arguments about that being another country, etc, and the numbers speak for themselves. Most of all, believe in yourself!

Alana, 25, Cork

If that's what you want, go for it! Don't let anybody talk you out of it unless you're in doubt yourself. Try and talk to other women who've had a home birth.

B, 42, Cork

For More information on Home birth in Ireland, visit the Home Birth Association of Ireland website at www.home birth.ie

Chapter Six

THE FOURTH TRIMESTER

"In the midst of my hormone crazed days, I wished for someone to tell me what to eat, what to wear, what to do. Eventually, that feeling passed too. Instead of looking at the big picture I started to take things day by day - sometimes moment by moment. I'd lie in bed with her and tell myself, "I am a mother. I have kept her alive despite those idiots at the hospital letting me take her home with no basic training whatsoever. It will be OK."

Cass, 43, Carlow

Wanted: Sleep. Will pay good money.

It's official. My children hate me. For what seems like the millionth night in a row, I have failed to achieve anything more than a "light doze" at any given point throughout the night. This, of course, does not include the coma I eventually fall into five minutes before the alarm goes off and the endless loop that is now my life begins anew.

The small one is at the peak - I hope, dear god I hope this is the peak!- of her "fussy" period. This is a time I had forgotten about. A time marked by constant feeding, grizzling and general irritation when they seem to be on a permanent growth spurt and the best advice that anyone can come up with is that, "This too shall pass..." (Thanks Chris!) The fussy period generally coincides with the eruption of infant acne which means that your angry red infant is now an angry, red, spotty infant.

Surely her big sister could never have gone through such a hideous phase! Surely I'd have remembered it and solemnly vowed never to procreate again!

Well, it seems Mother Nature (that canny ol'bitch) has a lot to answer for. You know that hormone that makes us forget exactly how bad labour was - or at least to remember it in soft focus? A similar process seems to be at work for the first few months of infant-hood as my mother assures me that yes, Lily did go through this and that yes, I did call her at 2:00a.m in an effort to save my sanity and prevent her granddaughter from being sold to the highest bidder.

Well, after this last week, I am on the verge of GIVING our newest arrival to anyone who will take her (and of course return her safe and sound when this "fussy" period ends and the infant acne clears.)

To add insult to injury, she has the most efficient digestive system I've ever seen which means that after she finishes devouring the contents of my breasts, all it takes is a quick flip to the upright position to produce a man sized burp followed by the ejection of any and all excess milk from her tummy. Said excess milk generally ends up coating whoever is unlucky enough to be holding her.

The remainder of her meals are then forcefully expelled into an increasingly messy series of curry colored nappies, the majority of which immediately leak onto my lap and/or the furniture.

So why do we persist? Why, if the tiny terrors are so blatantly antisocial, are the classifieds not filled with "free to good home" ads for wayward infants?

Because Mother Nature has yet another trick up her sleeve. Just as the gassiness, crying and general irritability reach their peak, just as their little eyes cross with the effort of expelling yet another high velocity poo, just as you realize you literally have NOTHING to wear that is not covered in some form of bodily fluid, just as you reach the end of your rope and are about to let go...They smile.

A great big, googly eyed, off kilter gummy grin that reaches in and grabs you by the heart, giving you the strength to get through yet another sleepless night.

Survival of the cutest. Infant Darwinism at it's finest.

Right, I'm off for my nap now

Real Mams Talk About:
The Early Days
If I'm totally honest, it was a bit of a shock the first time round - and a bit depressing at times! The hardest part was the loneliness. There were days when I would have paid someone just to sit at the kitchen table, talking wasn't necessary - I just wanted someone there with me! It felt like Groundhog Day, day after day... I lived for the weekends just to have my husband home with me. I used to pace the floor in the sitting room of an evening but it wasn't him I was waiting for, it was an extra pair of arms to hold the baby. When he used to ring me to say he was popping out to my mother's for a coffee before he headed on home, I used to say, "Okay, see you soon!" But inside I was thinking, "You fucker! Come home and you can have your coffee here! I need you to give me a break!" Don't get me wrong, I enjoyed motherhood (mostly) but there were days when I cried more than the baby did. My husband would be going down the stairs at seven a.m on his way to work and I'd be snot crying before he even reached the front door.

Gwen, Kildare

I remember coming home from the hospital and being so relieved that I could leave my son in one room and I could walk into another and I was no longer the person who was solely responsible for him. I hated the fact that I had to stay in the hospital and my husband could leave at nine pm and go for a pint! The biggest shock had to be the fact that a baby could take up all, and I mean ALL of your day. Countless cups of tea were left around with one mouthful taken out of them. If you had a shower, it was a great day and if you could make it till your husband came home without crying, well then! You were mother of the year material!

A, 33, Dublin

The early days of motherhood were amazing (as they still are). She is one of the happiest, smiliest, friendliest babies I have ever seen/known. Everyone comments on how smiley she is. She has been such a good baby from the start so we both took to parenthood like ducks to water. I think it also helped that we are that bit older and would be used to babies, what with looking after nieces and nephews, so there was no big shocks for us. Everyone said to get ready for the sleepless nights, but they never really came. For the first six weeks, she woke for a feed at two a.m (ish) and that was it till early morn! After that, with the exception of the odd dodgy night she slept all night every night!

Ruth, 36

It was very overwhelming, knowing that this little person was my sole responsibility. The day my partner went back to work, Amy cried all day long. Nothing I could do would satisfy her. It took a few days for me to realize that women have done this for hundreds of years and I was well able to do it also.

Jennifer, 28, Meath

I absolutely loved those first few days. I was smitten and couldn't take my eyes off of Clodagh. That even included throughout the night so therefore, I was very tired. The biggest shock was the realization that she would be depending on us as her parents for many years to come and hoping I would live up to the job.

Ingrid, 29, Cavan

They were an absolute horror to be honest. Everything was lovely in the hospital. Breast feeding was going grand, there were no sore nipples and I had a sleeping, eating, pooing baby with no crying. Then we came home... The crying never stopped and no one could tell us what was wrong. My hormones were crazy but I didn't dare show it! Top end sore, bottom end sore, trapped on the one chair from morning till night as everything melded into one. I remember sitting down looking at the TV with my husband and it was just snow and we didn't even notice. Then of course, we had everyone saying to us not to lift a crying baby as that will spoil it. We left him to cry for fifteen minutes once and I couldn't take it any longer. I lifted him up and he was wet through with sweat. I'm still traumatized by the memory. You CANNOT spoil a baby that small and when this next one arrives, I'll use the baby sling a lot more if I have to.

Margaret, 34, Louth

To be honest, the early days were awful. I knew they would be but nothing prepares you for it. I thought rooming in was awful. I really think if I'd had even three or four hours on my own I would have been much more rested and prepared, but I got no rest at all and literally thought I was going to die with exhaustion. I had very low blood pressure and was having dizzy spells. I kept thinking I was going to collapse and half hoping I would so that someone would feel sorry for me and help me out! Although I'd never even seen a newborn, let alone held one, I was surprisingly comfortable with my son. It helped that he was a massive, fat 9lb 11oz baby. It just felt natural. I can't say that I felt that rush of love you hear about, but I certainly felt fiercely protective of him and got a bit jealous when visitors passed him around.

Laura, 30, Cork

My Mum came to stay for a few days, my husband stayed home from work for the next few and then...Nothing !! It was like jumping into the arctic ocean, two babies, one aged 12.5 months, one just a week old... OH MY GOD !

Ciara, 33, Dublin

Becoming Mammy

I became a mother the day my daughter was conceived. I became a mammy about five years later. I did not enjoy my pregnancy. I did not glow and my feet got to the point where a shoe box and a bit of elastic would have been preferable to the expandable sandals which left a pressure callous on my foot only an angle grinder could remove.

When my breasts were measured, the woman announced my size and I thought she said eye, not I. Good God! How did I become an I Cup?!?!?!? People pay big money for measurements like that! My waist went from a curvy thirty two to a more circular fifty six. I felt like one of those "roly poly won't fall down" dolls.

How do you glow when every time you get up you are beaten back by your own monstrous breasts? How do you "radiate" when your feet look like they are about to explode?

My husband was afraid. When I demanded - yes demanded - a blue Mr. Freeze in February, he scoured the county and came back with a bag full of offerings - none of which were blue - and was rewarded for his efforts with a mere grunt.

When my due date came around, I had to have a c section. I am by no means an earth mother and I did not feel cheated by missing out on the opportunity to try and push a child from a place I can barely remove a tampon from at the best of times. My vagina is not unlike Irish roads - sharp bends ahead.

When my daughter was born, she was as yellow as a turnip and had to be put under the lights. The midwives asked, did I not want to go and visit her? I looked at them as if they were mad. I had just had five layers of flesh cut open. I had a rash in places I hadn't looked at in months that was driving me around the twist. My feet were like water balloons and they wanted me to trudge upstairs to visit the small one who'd been leasing my uterus for the last nine months. She and I had been together for long enough, surely I deserved a bit of a kip!

I didn't say it though. Instead I went up the stairs to her and it was like this little alien, I knew it was mine but cripes, what was I supposed to do? I was very resentful for awhile. Everybody came to see the baby. There I was - bloody, cut up, feet swollen, covered in hives, bawling my eyes out - and nobody seemed at all interested. My last childish temper tantrum I suppose.

When the daughter was seven hours old she had her first temper tantrum. I wheeled her to the nursery and requested an anger management class for the baby. They thought I was mad. How was I to know that babies are not just peeing, pooping, eating, sleeping, puking machines? That they develop a personality from your input, love and guidance.

I just thought, "Oh crap what have I done?"

My perception of what a mother was changed so much in those first four hours. She taught me that there would always be a war of wills and that my job would be to figure out the difference between the needs and the wants. I got out the books for help and then threw them away because they did not seem to have a grasp on my screaming poop pot.

When it came to breastfeeding she did not take to it for ten weeks. I was determined though as I have severe allergies and hoped this would diminish the possibility of her inheriting them. Finally, I had to buy a pump. Not just a single either, but a double. My husband says he can still hear the whir of the pump in his memory and see the image of his beloved hooked up like a heifer in his mind's eye.

He eventually had to request a new storage method for the milk though, when he accidentally used it in his tea. I never thought

I would see the day when there was a jar labeled, " Today's breast milk," in my fridge.

It wasn't until I'd spent a small fortune on bottles that my daughter finally learned how to breast feed. After that, she didn't leave me alone for years. She could smell my milk a mile away and she'd start making this sucking sound. It was like having my very own, very small stalker.

My wardrobe changed. I hated women who were all done up as my clothes had to be stain resistant with easy breast access. Shoes were no longer chosen for style but for comfort and as I was incontinent half the time I had to wear black so it could not be seen. At one point I thought it would be clever to cut my hair in what was little more then a buzz cut as it would mean less hair to wash.

Not a good move, I looked like a mad woman.

I couldn't wear thongs; piles put an end to that. Had I thought that a large flap of skin protruding over a lovely, lacy pair of underpants would be in any way attractive, I would not have resorted to cotton granny pants.

Even the bath wasn't safe. Fat floats, and having to face piggy feet, fat flaps and leaky breasts was not my idea of a great way to relax. Bubbles became my best friend.

I used to fantasize about smothering my husband. He would sleep, while the stalker was after me. He didn't have to learn the skill of catching puke while driving or have involuntary bodily changes and mood swings. He didn't get any, "I am only suggesting...." advice from helpful friends, family and passersby. He did not have to panic when our darling daughter drank the floor cleaner, pulled the dresser over on herself, or when she turned blue trying to win the eating war.

In the midst of my hormone crazed days, I wished for someone to tell me what to eat, what to wear, what to do. Eventually, that feeling passed too. Instead of looking at the big picture I started to take things day by day - sometimes moment by moment. I'd lie in bed with the stalker and tell myself, "I am a mother. I have kept her alive despite those idiots at the hospital letting me take her home with no basic training whatsoever. It will be OK."

I fed and washed her. I did all the things I was meant to do as a mother, but it wasn't until when in a medical situation she looked to me for reassurance, that I truly felt like a mammy. I realized then, that all of the things I had thought were important, were not nearly as important as our daughter feeling safe in our arms.

At last, with that trust and re-assurance came that deep, primal feeling.

I had the glow thing at about three months. You know, awe and all that stuff, but the connection wasn't really there. We have a relationship now. I love to watch her grow, her laughter fills my heart. When she achieves something she thought she could not do, I am her cheerleader. I love to see her develop into the wonderful person she is. I wish I had not been so scared. I wish I had not been so caught up in doing everything by the book and in trying to please everyone and caring what they all thought just because I got a little bit lost.

At the end of the day, you instill in your children respect for themselves and for others along with the other basic life lessons. Don't pick your nose and eat it. No, the cat would not like a bath. Corn belongs in your mouth not your nose.

And then one day you wake up and find that that body destroying stalker is a really neat person and you can't imagine your life without them.

We, herself and myself, just spent five solid weeks together in my home country, Canada. It was there that I realized that I am an Irish mammy. I indulge with sweets. We have ice cream on a cold winters day. We pack picnics for the big train ride. Dear God, I'd have it no other way.

My skin flaps are a testament to it. I stand proud in my micro fiber re-enforced smalls, stain resistant wash and wear garments, elastic side strap shoes and out of control hair.

I know how to live now, moment by moment and making the most of them all. Never feeling so complete as when in the arms of a child because you make them feel secure and loved.

That's a mammy to me.

Cass, 43, Carlow

Real Mams Talk About:
Your Body After Birth

It is a real shock that your body takes a long time to get back to normal. And really that's a new normal, because for me, once I had a baby, my body never went back to the way it was before. My whole shape had changed. I have certain jeans and trousers, and I know that no matter how much weight I lose, I will never get back into them. People talked to me about six weeks being a big landmark and it was really. At that stage you can walk with the buggy and not feel exhausted.

A, 33, Dublin

SKINNY, SKINNY, SKINNY. After the birth I was 1.5 stone lighter than BEFORE I got pregnant. I was in better shape after the birth than I had been in about 3 years. I felt better than myself. I was so astonished. I'm not a small girl, regularly size 14-16, and prone to putting on weight if I don't watch myself. I assumed I would balloon when I was pregnant, but the opposite happened. I lost a stone and a half and put it back on while pregnant, then was a stone and a half lighter when

Izzy arrived......brilliant way for me to lose weight, completely unexpected!!

Karen, 29

Jelly Belly, it just wobbled around!!!! I breast fed my first, and was back into my own clothes in no time, about five weeks I think. With Joanne, I breast fed for four weeks, and definitely think it helped, but I had to work harder to get any shape back. Walking was definitely the best thing I did. Both my babies started sleeping through the night at about nine weeks, and that is when I really started to feel like myself again.

Christine, 29, Wicklow

Back in shape????? She is five months old and I'm not in shape. Nine months on, nine months off. Don't rush yourself. My body was sore after the birth. My scar healed well but getting the staples out wasn't nice. I felt like myself after about a few weeks of adjusting.

Leanne, 26, Dublin

On my first, I was thinner after I had my baby then I was before because I had the morning sickness so bad for six months. I felt great! On my second, I gained over a stone which I found hard to lose. I still haven't lost it in fact. So I will have to work doubly hard after this one. I'm not too bothered about it to be honest. There are now more important things in my life to worry about than my body.

Elaine, 29, Cork

Wobbly...and leaky! My belly felt like play dough and my arse was fat. I remember a friend asking me how it all felt down below and I said 'It feels like my crank shaft has fallen out.' Now I don't know what a crank shaft is of even if it exists but if it did, it would be important! In February, I just thought 'right enough of this' and booked into the hairdressers. I went from long and darkish to short and blonde. And I started Pilates. I just felt like I needed to get back to me. The funny thing is, is that the old me NEVER exercised!

Kirsty, 29

To say I felt battered and bruised was an understatement! After having the episiotomy I was very, very uncomfortable and I never thought I would get back to normal. But after a few weeks, the stitches dissolved and I never thought I'd be so happy to be able to sit properly again! I was in no hurry to lose my baby weight and hadn't thought about exercising but gradually, with eating little and often and getting as much sleep as I can when baby is resting I'm starting to feel like my old self again.

Kim, 22, Dublin

I felt great after two weeks when the stitches stopped hurting because that was so sore. If I had escaped stitches, I would have been great after three days!

Fiona, 28, Kildare

A wibbly wobbly wonder that still passed gas without warning!

Gwen

I'm not sure if this happens after a section or birth in general but my whole body swelled up like a balloon especially my feet which was very scary. I wear size eight shoes as it is so I was hoping they wouldn't stay that big. Also, after day three, my milk supply came in and that was painful. My boobs were huge and rock hard. I was leaking liters every morning which was very embarrassing. Luckily I was in the hospital for six days as Clodagh had to go into Special care as she was jaundiced so I was able to get plenty of help and advice from the Lactation Expert on relieving the pain.

Ingrid, 29, Cavan

Sore boobs, bum, piles, stitches, achy belly......hard to walk!! That all took about three to six weeks to get back to normal down there! Although six months on and my body seems to have changed for good :-(Droopy boobs and stretch marks aren't pretty!

Jane, 32, Dublin

I had a sixteen hour labour that ended with ventouse and forceps being used. I tore badly and ended up in surgery for two and a half hours after Amy was born. I was in an awful state. It took me four to six weeks before I could walk for any length of time without wincing and eleven months later I'm still two stone overweight, although that is my fault and not pregnancy's!

Jennifer, 29, Meath

I feel like a car crash victim. Seven weeks later and I'm slowly getting back to resembling a functioning person. It's not so bad after natural births, they were definitely easier to recover from.

Jennifer, 33, Dublin

Hmmm, smaller, wobbly, sore, tired, leaky, cracked nipples, tender.

Jenny, Cork

It never really did get back into the shape it was before, because I didn't make much of an effort for it to. I didn't start feeling like myself until I stopped breastfeeding at four months and could wear normal under-wire bras and t shirts and not be worrying about leaky boobs and nursing tops.

Lara, 28, Meath

Flabby, sore, achy, heavy, unsexy, used, ugly, empty, not mine!

Samantha

My body still isn't in proper shape. Now, don't get me wrong. I was never a size zero but I am a fourteen now when I was always a twelve! I can't seem to get rid of my jelly belly (always had a belly but not quite as big as it is now) To be honest, it's worth it. I'm happy having a stretch marked jelly belly.

Ruth, 36, Dublin

Weak, bloated, gross, unfamiliar, traumatized, exhausted, womanly, amazing, natural, fulfilled. The last few are positive, because although I felt and looked horrendous, I couldn't believe that this body gave life to something so wonderful. It was a great feeling.

Laura, 30, Cork

Gwen's Advice to First Time Mothers

My advice to first time mams is... Don't listen to any advice! In order to do this you must not tell people the truth. About anything! If your baby roars his head off day and night, smile brightly through the red mist floating in front of your eyes and tell people he is a good little sleeper. He probably is once he drops off, it's just getting him there is the problem. So you're not really lying.

Much...

Everybody has advice but nobody has the correct solution to this particular problem.

While we're on the subject, there is no magic way to make your baby sleep "through the night" by the time they're six weeks old. They will do this when they are ready. By the way, sleeping through and sleeping the night are two completely different things. Sleeping through means going for five or six hours between feeds which, if your baby is asleep for ten pm, means that you will still be getting up at three am. Again, lie and tell people your baby sleeps twenty four/seven. This will come in handy when they start talking about the four hourly thing.

whispers it isn't a crime if your baby doesn't do this either.

There is also this rumor doing the rounds that there will be a big difference when your baby is three months old. Basically, if your baby is still crying round the clock, not sleeping and has colic after this coming of age, you will wonder (a) what's wrong with him? or (b) what's wrong with YOU?

By the same token, your baby needs to be fed one way or the other. It is up to you how you decide to feed your baby, you don't need to explain to people why you choose to breast or bottle feed. Or choose to breastfeed past a certain age.

Don't allow anyone to make you doubt how you want to respond to your child. If, like me, you're happy to comfort him if he's caught his finger in a door or just toppled over and wants a cuddle, CUDDLE HIM! Yes, he'll be alright, but he'll be even better and better quicker in his mammy's arms!

If you're not happy to have your baby cry, pick him up. No-one's baby was ever removed from their care for loving them too much! You can only love a baby too little.

In a nut shell, you have to be able to function the next day and if keeping your baby in your bed at night enables you to do this, then so be it. Just sssshhhh! Don't tell anyone!

It's pretty easy for those who have enjoyed a full and uninterrupted eight hours of sleep, to have the answer to our babies sleep problems. I don't know if it's the sight of them sitting here with their legs and arms crossed that annoys me most or the fact that they are about to finish one of many cups of tea without having to get up to wipe a snotty nose or remove a dangerous object from little hands!

Naturally I'd advise you not to take any of this advice as you will find your own sweet way as you plod along and before you know it, you'll be coming up with pearls of wisdom yourself!

Gwen, Kildare

Real Mams Talk About:
Advice to New Mams...

Ha Ha!! The first thing I would tell anyone to do is to throw away all the baby books!! I threw the GF one in the bin, cos she scared the life out of me with her routines - left boob ten minutes, right boob ten minutes. I mean, come on! They're babies, not soldiers. THEY ARE ALL DIFFERENT! Another thing would be not to believe mothers who tell you that their babies sleep through the night - they are lying, or else they have a very different definition to yours as to what constitutes sleeping through the night.

Always trust your instinct. No one knows your baby like you do and that includes doctors. If you think that there is something not right, persist. A good Doctor will always listen to a parent.

Another thing to remember is that things do get better - the baby gets into a routine, you get to have a shower on a daily basis and eventually, you do get your evenings back, hurrah!

Anon, 33, Dublin

You know what, I'd say it's okay to feel like absolute crap, like a failure and like asking, "Is there no way I can give this thing back?" Help! Book me a one way ticket to Australia! Yes, some people are just blown away with love and affection and happy out all the time from the first second, but there are just as many people who feel that this is bloody hard work, place far too high expectations on themselves and are gutted when the fairy tale doesn't happen. I feel so passionate about this. Women owe it to women to be honest, but then again, maybe we just don't listen when we are told, cruel Mother Nature!

Joanne, 35, Kerry

What do I wish I'd been told? That it is hard work, that babies cry a lot, that your relationship with your husband will never be the same again, that you will feel guilty and inadequate all the time and that no matter what you read your baby will not conform to the standards. That night feeds are always hard, that exhaustion is like an illness, that even women who appear as if they are together are finding it tough and that no matter how much you love them there are days when you just wish you had never even had sex in the first place.

Amber, 36, Cork

Don't expect too much from yourself and make sure your partner understands this too. I was beating myself up for not being able to do everything and unfortunately there was no one in my life who could tell me that I needed to slow down. I felt I wasn't organized enough and was always struggling but looking back, I did so much in those first few weeks, I was out and about almost immediately and traveling with my baby at just a few weeks old. I was really stressed and felt that there was something lacking in me but now I realize that I was just trying to do too much too soon.

Don't expect family and friends to understand how your life has changed unless they have been there. Go to support groups to meet other new mums as they are the only ones who can understand you. Don't let yourself feel isolated or stressed alone.

Anon, 31, Cork

I wish people had told me that it's okay to admit to being bored when you're on maternity leave. It doesn't mean that you don't love your new baby or that you don't want to spend all your time with them. However, if you're living somewhere with no friends or family close by and no means of transport to get you places, then you can feel isolated and then guilty for feeling that just being with your baby is not company enough.

Lara, 28, Meath

Firstly, enjoy your pregnancy if possible. Sleep while you can because it will be a precious commodity in the first few months. Be prepared for a messy house and little or no time to tidy it. To this day an untidy house really gets me down and I find it very hard to get time to do anything about it and if I do, it's usually undone for me in about an hour or two! I suppose support is a major factor also. Tell your hubby/partner that you are going to need him on board 100% and make sure he is agreeable, although in my case he was totally up for it but when it came to the crunch it all fell back on me, both the day to day care of the kids and all the housework.

Louise, 28, Cavan

Take all the help you are offered and all the second hand stuff you can get. Bin the books, apart from the totally practical ones. Trust your instincts. Shut the door - or more politely your ears - to people who use the words "you should," or "baby should." "Should" is the most stressful word a new mam can hear. Take advice that suits you and ignore the rest, however well-intentioned it may be!

Chris, 31, Cork

This could be long winded! I wish someone had told me honestly that sleep deprivation is hell...That I could've bought lots of things second hand to save money...That yes, you really can breastfeed after a section...That my husband would put so much pressure on me to know what was wrong with our baby. He needed to ask me EVERYTHING!!! I wish for the first few months that I had relaxed and trusted my own instincts and not worried that I was a crap mother cos I couldn't do fifty million things all at once! I wish that I had not let everyone hold my baby when he was a day old as it made him very unsettled and it wasn't fair on him. The main thing really, is that I should've just trusted my own judgement in situations and not let people like my mother make me feel bad for decisions I make as Conor's mum. I will know better for next time.

Emma, 29, Cork

I got, read (and re-read), all of the pregnancy books, looking for some way to bond with my little man, as I couldn't hold him, but as for the parenting in the first year books ... Well, lets just say that I've offered them to anyone who will have them. I genuinely thought everything that was written in them was a whole load of pig manure. I don't want to hear about what age he should be doing what at. What people need is a book that will tell you tried and tested ways of dealing with teething, nappy rash, colds and general everyday things as tried by real mothers.

Laura, 23, Tipperary

Well Laura! Since you asked...

Practical Advice on the Day to Day Running of Your Baby
Don't waste a fortune on a super duper travel system buggy, they are too big and bulky, and you only use them for a few months anyway. You don't need every baby book going, and no one can give you better advice than a fellow mum. If you need advice on anything, go to a library to borrow a book, or better still, use a website such as rollercoaster.ie or magicmum.ie

Christine, 29, Wicklow

I read a lot of books but actually ended up doing it my own way. I nursed her all the time and fed her on demand. She slept through the night from three weeks. I had her in our bed with us for the first while. Don't try and force routine too early. Everything is new to this little person. It'll take them a while to get their bearings.

Leanne, 26, Donegal

After my first child was born, I was exhausted. People would appear unannounced on the door step to see the baby, expecting tea and biscuits, and stay for ages! Being so tired, I didn't have the strength to ask them to leave. On my second, I made sure that people rang before calling in, and if they did just appear, I was able to ask them to leave once I had "had enough." I knew that being tired and having sleepless nights was part of it, but I didn't realize just how tiring it all was.

Christine, 29, Wicklow

Don't whisper around a sleeping baby. Noise equals a relaxed atmosphere!

Jane, 32, Dublin

I totally recommend a routine from as early as possible. We muddled through with no set bedtime and demand feeding for the first four months and I was absolutely shattered. Myself and my husband had no time for a chat in the evenings at all. At four months, we moved our baby into her own room, put her on four hourly feeds, and started a proper bed time routine with a bath and story. We have never looked back as from then on she has slept all night. We are early risers so she gets up at seven each day and she goes to bed at eight, leaving us with a lovely long evening together which is very important.

Ingrid, 29, Cavan

I found cabbage leaves from the fridge great for breast feeding when they got a little full.

Elaine, 29, Cork

Regarding quick meals, there is absolutely nothing wrong with having a back-up supply of spaghetti hoops and the likes in your cupboard for those days when you just could not be bothered cooking! Also pancakes and drop scones are really quick and easy as well. I graduated from "The Cheats School of Cooking" sometime back in 2007!!

Gwen, Kildare,

This sounds mad but the Lactation expert in the hospital gave me a great tip for engorged breasts that really works. Get two nappies and run the absorbent side under really hot water and wring out excess water. Then place them onto your breasts and fasten the sticky tape. The heat really helps to express the pressure of excess milk.

Ingrid, 29, Cavan

Make sure to wash and dry your baby's folds everyday! It's amazing how much crap gets stuck in them and they get irritated so fast with all the drool. If they do get a bit weepy, try a bit of sudocrem to keep infection at bay.

P, Dublin

For nappy rash, nappy free time. The open air will help it heal very quickly. Also, I NEVER used creams on Ger's bottom. A friend of mine used them from the day her kids were born, and they've always had sore bums. And most of all, you can't beat cotton wool and water after a pooh in the early weeks.

Laura, 23, Tipperary

The one tip l have to give other new mammies is to try doing the 'dreamfeed' it's the most amazing thing to watch and although my little one wouldn't do it till she was five or six weeks old, it worked perfectly till we dropped it when she was around seven months. Other new parents we have spoken to were going on about how they woke their baby for the 11:00pm feed and sometimes ended up with them awake till the early hours of the morning. When we told them about the dreamfeed it totally changed everything and being up half the night was no longer a problem. Apart from this l have no other words of wisdom....

Ruth, 36, Dublin

Sing, sing, sing... music and songs are so much fun and then when baby falls a familiar song will pull them right out of their misery.

Ciara, 33, Dublin

Breast milk is magic stuff! My little one suffered with recurring sticky eye (conjunctivitis) for the first seven months of her life as her tear ducts were too small and needed time to properly develop. A few drops of milk in the eye a few times a day worked a charm whenever her eyes were acting up!

Jess, Galway

Own brand nappies are just as good if not better then the big brands and only a fraction of the price. Your baby doesn't care what brand he's wearing so long as you change him regularly!

Emily, 27, Tipperary

For really bad nappy rash, try making a nappy cake. One layer of sudocreme followed by a layer of baby powder or corn starch and then another layer of cream. Works every time.

Ger, Mam of 4, Waterford

If you're having trouble getting your baby to settle, turn on the extractor fan and then walk around the room with them until they settle. The fan acts like white noise and knocks them out cold!

Jen, 32, Kildare

For a snuffly nose, those snot bulb things (I forget their name) and a drop of saline spray give instant relief. Also, if your breastfeeding, nurse as much as your baby wants when their sick because every time you latch your baby on, you give them the benefit of your own antibodies to fight off whatever it is that's bothering them.

Claire, Mam of Two, Kilkenny

Invest in a sling. They're super handy and babies love them. Your baby is happy snuggled up next to mum and you have your arms free to do what you like! Go to the Babywearing Ireland website and talk to the mums there. There is so much research about the benefits of wearing your baby and I can honestly say that the bloody thing saved my sanity! I never had one on my first as it was a little too "hippy" for me but I got one on my second and have never looked back. There are sling libraries all over Ireland where you can try out slings to see which ones suit you best as there are so many types on offer and the big shops only tend to carry the more mainstream carrier types which aren't that good for baby's spine in the first few months. It's all on the babywearing site though, so check it out. I can't recommend them highly enough.

Trish, 37, Cavan

Keep two sets of change gear (nappies, wipes, onesies etc...) One for upstairs and one for down. We never bothered with a big change table, just kept everything in two Tupperware boxes and had 2 portable change mats so we could throw him down wherever we happened to be.

Mam of Three, Meath

Don't be afraid to give cloth nappies a go! The ones for sale nowadays are a far cry from the terry nappies and plastic pants of old and come in all different price ranges. Even if you get the most expensive ones out there, you'll still save a bundle in the long run. Research the different types and maybe do a trial of a few different makes to see what works for you. You can make your own wipes as well by ripping up one of those fleece blankets you get at Penny's or Dunnes for a fiver and soaking them in a little plastic box with cool boiled water and a few drops of lavender oil. Have a look on line at the on line parenting sites to find other mums who use them. They're full of advice and you can often grab some second hand deals as well!

Lisa, 31, Limerick

Four in the Bed

When I was pregnant on my first child, I had very definite ideas on how my baby would be raised. Co Sleeping did not figure highly in these plans.

In fact, it didn't figure at all. As far as I was concerned, our baby would be sleeping in a cot, in its own room, from day one. I had read Gina Ford, well, skimmed... okay, I read the introduction where I was promised a perfectly timed eating, sleeping, pooping, contented little baby and then threw it aside to be dealt with later.

At the time, it made sense to me. Babies were brand new people unaccustomed to the ways and means of our world. It was our job as parents to train them in these ways. They needed cots and nurseries, black out blinds and white noise machines. Above all else though, they needed ROUTINE.

Yes, that great, oft repeated word from every baby book ever written and whispered into the sweet shell like ears of new mothers all over the western world. Routine, like Jesus and low fat cheese spread, would save us all.

What I hadn't planned on was a week's stay in hospital after the baby was born. A week where night after night, my new little citizen would scream the ward down if I so much as pointed her in the direction of her plastic bassinet. It was on or around the fourth night of our stay that one of the midwives suggested I take her into the bed with me.

A week earlier, I'd have looked at her like she was insane and reported her for negligence. Good Lord! I had enough trouble with the concept of the baby in our room, let alone in our bed!

It's amazing what a little sleep deprivation will do to those hard set ideals.

It was the best. Night's. Sleep. Ever.

For the rest of my stay, myself and the tiny being who would eventually become known as the snot queen, slept cocooned together in my fuzzy red housecoat. Day and night, her warm little body would lie curled against me, rising and falling with every breath.

Once home, she spent a few nights in a Moses basket next to our bed. She hated the basket though and as it was I would invariably doze off during the night feed and wake up with her still in my arms.

We tried a cot with the same result, thinking maybe it was space she craved. It wasn't though, it was us. By the end of month two, "Our Bed" officially became "The Family Bed" and I became extremely well read on the subject of co sleeping and its many benefits.

I experienced for myself how much easier it made breastfeeding and would often wake to find she had latched on and fed while I was asleep.

When I found out I was pregnant on number two, friends and family who were "concerned" about our sleeping arrangements started making helpful suggestions about how the Snot Queen would have to be moved into a bed of her own and how the new baby should really learn to sleep in a cot.

We nodded and smiled and listened politely to everything they said.

In the end, we got a bigger bed.

Real Mams Talk About:
Co sleeping

My sister and brother-in-law have always had a family bed and my parents had my sister and I in the room with them when we were little, so it always seemed very natural to me. When my little girl was born, I couldn't imagine having her in this plastic cot when she could be warm and cosy next to me and close to her food supply. We had a co sleeper bed purchased and some nights the baby was in that and other nights she was between my husband and I, whichever was the most comfortable and convenient. It wasn't until after we had begun co sleeping that I started to research and see the benefits and how it could reduce the chance of cot death and also was so much easier to breast-feed during the night.

Erin, 31, Cork

Decision was reached by accident. Our daughter, as someone said, opened a can of whoop-ass on us and would not sleep in a cot. The only place she slept was next to us. And then we liked it, and we all got some sleep. She came into bed day one at home. Daughter number two came into the bed in the hospital!

Mairead

It happened in the hospital. When we got home I did not even raise it with my husband. It was the one thing he was adamant about before we gave birth. Poor man, I had put him through enough of my "alternative" ways up to now, this was a bridge too far for him. Well we put her in the moses basket beside us. She cried for five minutes and he said put her in the bed. We have never looked back. She slept with us until she moved into her "big girls bed" bed at a year and a half.

Now my hubby has become one of those daddy bores and tells anyone who will listen that he can't understand why anyone would not at least want mom and baby in the same bed – sure mom has carried baby in her tummy for 9 ½ months. That is 9 ½ months of mommy's heart beat, voice, smell etc... He thinks and says to anyone who will listen that it is the most natural extension of this and the most natural place for babies to be.

Cita, Kildare

It was a very conscious decision for us to co sleep. I read a lot about it before she was born, and we decided to get a bigger bed instead of a cot. We were all ready for her when she was born. Day one, she slept beside us in a snuggle nest as I was too tired to trust myself after labour. Since day two, she just sleeps between us in bed. Because it was a conscious decision I was able to get all the things I needed to make the bed and bedclothes safe.

Alana, 25, Cork

(Author's note: If you are considering co sleeping with your child/children, please do your research first and look into safe co sleeping practices. A full list of safety precautions can be found at www.drsears.com *Never, under any circumstances, co sleep with your baby while under the influence of drugs, alcohol or any substance which may cause you to sleep heavier then normal.)*

Chapter Seven

BREASTFEEDING IN IRELAND: PART ONE

Realizing that we as mothers are made to nourish our babies physically and emotionally is very empowering and I personally feel honored to have that privilege. I know that it can be challenging at times but can only say that it is so very worth it. Few things are insurmountable and I wouldn't change a moment of those challenges for they make me value the wonderful nursing relationship I have with my now eighteen month old daughter all the more. There's so much more to it than milk!

Kara

Breastfeeding: What's Normal?

Well, for starters, Breastfeeding is normal. It isn't "Best," or "exceptional" or even "Supreme." It's normal. It isn't "Vulgar," "Gross" or "Obscene" either. It's normal. It doesn't make you a better person or a better mother. You don't get extra club card points for doing it.

You're baby is not shocked when you latch him on for the first feed. This isn't some sort of treat, it's what he was expecting. In fact, any newborn, when lain on the mother's tummy immediately after birth and left to their own devices, will automatically make their way to the breast and latch on. Why? Because it's what babies have done since the dawn of humanity. This is nothing new. In fact, it even has a name. It's called the breast crawl. You can look it up if you like.

As for the milk itself, again, nothing special, just the same old milk that human mothers have always made for human babies. They haven't changed the recipe. It doesn't give your child super powers or make them "better," or "exceptional," in any way. Just normal.

You don't believe me? Let's have a look at it, shall we?

First we have colostrum, the sticky yellow stuff that gets produced towards the end of pregnancy and in the first days after birth. It's full of the same old antibodies and proteins that give the baby passive immunity while his own immune system is still maturing and helps the digestive system to grow and develop like normal.

You see? Normal! Not better, just normal, the way it's designed to work. It also acts as a mild laxative to help get the meconium (your baby's black, tarry first poo) out and keep all of that bilirubin (you know, the stuff that can contribute to jaundice) from building up. Again, nothing new here! Moving on, we have the more mature milk, that whitish stuff we're more familiar with that comes in around the second or third day.

It's still made up of fore milk and hind milk. Fore milk being the sweet, watery, almost bluish stuff that comes out at the start of a feed and quenches the babies thirst before it changes into the thicker, fattier, creamy stuff that fills them up and satisfies their hunger. It's still full of all the same old nutrients that the baby needs for normal growth and development. Nothing more, nothing less.

It provides that same link to the mother's immune system that it's always had. Again, what's new about that? It's called passive immunity and all it means is that as long as a child is being fed at the breast, they will receive their mother's antibodies against certain diseases and viruses via the breast milk until their own immune system is mature and can produce antibodies of its own.

Do you want me to continue? Because I can. I can tell you about how the composition of a mother's milk changes as her baby grows to suit his needs as a toddler and not just as an infant. I can tell you about how our babies learn new tastes by the subtle changes of flavor that our milk undergoes depending on what we eat. I can tell you about that wonderful hormone that helps mum go back to sleep after a middle of the night feed and baby to do the same. I could go on and on and on... but really, what would be the point? It's human milk.

It's no different now then it always has been. They haven't even bothered to change the packaging! I mean, come on...

Breastfeeding, what's the big deal?

It's normal.

Jenna's Story

I was 22 when my first son arrived. I was determined to breast feed. Not for any particular reason other than I was breastfed, and I felt that this is the way it was supposed to be. It became more important when he was admitted into NICU and fought for his life.

I pumped religiously and finally got to feed him myself for the first time at four days old. It was painful. There was little guidance or information about latching on. I thought this was just the way it was. I knew I was doing the right thing, the healthy thing, so I struggled on.

He was 9lbs 8ozs at birth, and a hungry baby. I knew no different, so I fed him whenever he wanted it. The advice I was given from well meaning mothers, was that this child needs to fit into my life; my life cannot revolve around him. I thought this was good advice until I found myself resenting this tiny little body for needing me so much.

But is that not what being a Mother is all about? Satisfying the needs of this human being that is reliant on you? Once I overcame the expectation that my life wasn't supposed to change, I started to enjoy breastfeeding. It was so satisfying to know that I, and only I could give this little baby what he needed. I was his superhero! Most newborns don't show much personality in their first few weeks and it is hard to gauge what they are thinking and feeling. However there is no mistaking the joy when a drunken blissful milky face stares up at you after a feed. It melted my heart over and over again. He had cute little habits like stroking rhythmically from shoulder to shoulder. He would stick his hand in my mouth and play with my lips. Those tiny moments were mine! No one else's.

Baby number two came 18 months after my first. I was given plenty of attention to get her to latch properly and feed well. It was far easier than feeding my son. A number of factors combined to end breastfeeding for us. When she was two days old, I couldn't get her to settle at night. A midwife came in with a top up bottle. After 10mls she was fast asleep. I felt like a failure. 'See just that small few drops is all she needed' is what the midwife said to me. It was the beginning of the end.

I fed her for two months and take comfort in the fact that she got the first weeks of the good stuff! Between baby two and three I attended UCC and studied Early Childhood Studies. I nicknamed our Nutrition class my Bad Mommy Class. We were bombarded with studies of how breastfeeding for x amount of weeks provided protection against x y z diseases. I felt terrible that I hadn't persevered with my daughter and breast fed her for longer.

Baby number three arrived, and boy I was determined. I firmly refused top up bottles in hospital and let baby suckle for as long as she wanted. I worried that my milk was taking so long to come in, but I let her at it and our bodies finally synchronized. When she needed it, I had it. Now at ten months old, we are still going strong. In the early days, yes, feeding times were frequent, but nothing beats the satisfaction you get from that blissful sleepy face grinning at you after a feed.

I have loved the quiet time I have had with each of my kiddies. Breastfeeding for me has been a simple equation. They needed to be fed, and I could do it. There will come times in my children's lives, where I will not be enough, I will not be able to provide the help and protection they need. So, doing this small thing at the very beginning of their lives is the very least I can do, and I love it.

Mairead's Story

I decided to breastfeed because I've always thought, "What else would you do?" A week or two before I had G, I had read that 99% of Swedish women breastfed, so I thought, "shur why wouldn't I be able to breast feed?"

Isn't it the strangest thing that people think you might not be "able" to breastfeed. Every other mammal feeds their young without question.

Then at our antenatal classes we were advised to buy a box of formula. So I did as I was told, bought a box and started reading the ingredients. Have you ever read them? Holy mother! I wouldn't drink the stuff myself, how could I give it to a tiny baba? To me, breastfeeding seemed like the only thing to do. I didn't really think much more about it.

Then I had my baby and was completely unprepared for the thunderbolt of love that hit me when I clapped eyes on her. She was a good sucker, which was lucky, cos I found the support in the hospital poor enough, and confusing.

On day two or three, my daughter was a bit jaundiced and my nurse was quite stroppy about wanting to give her formula. I had a strong instinct to give her breast milk only, but it's such a vulnerable time. Thankfully, I managed to stick to my guns and of course my daughter was perfectly fine. She would - as we now know - have let us know if she wasn't.

What is the obsession with formula in this country? You would think it was amazing medicine the way people go on. Liquid gold. When really, what's liquid gold is breast milk.

So I arrived home, post-section, with my baby and cracked nipples. Toe-curling pain is how I described it. But I continued. G cried a lot. Fed or not, she cried. I had my suspicions. I thought she had reflux but we soldiered on. Nights were horrendous, days not much better. I was anemic and knackered.

At the public health nurse, I mentioned how I thought G had reflux, all the crying and you just could not lie her flat. I lay her down to demonstrate, G screamed. The nurse hmmm-ed a minute and then suggested that because I was an "older" mum, and that I had worked professionally for a good few years, that maybe I wasn't adjusting to life at home and the demands of a baby, maybe I was depressed. I told her I didn't think so, look, I can't lie her down. But that was that. Go home and give her a bottle.

I came home, sat with my husband and wondered, " Could I be depressed?"

I thought about it and decided no, I'm enjoying life, I'm delighted with my baby, I'm looking forward to everything. Then I thought about the "bottle" advice. I read the ingredients on the formula box again, why would I give her a bottle? Why would anyone give a bottle? I battled on for another four months, when she had food refusal and ended up dehydrated and in A+E for IV fluids.

Guess what? She was diagnosed with reflux. She started on Zantac and our lives were transformed. We had this very happy, content, chirpy baby after all. In short, I found medical support hopeless.

Family support was as good as working family support can be. I remember one sis once saying in response to my repeated woes of tiredness: "Well, if you DO insist on feeding her every feed yourself...." The implication being that I was fussing and should just give her the odd bottle of formula and get on with it. I never complained to her again, and in fairness to her, her outlook has changed a lot and she was a great support with my second daughter.

I had no idea how long I would feed. Occasionally it was "one more feed and that's it." But all of a sudden, G was four months, then six, and it was easier, and she was so happy and I loved feeding her, so I kept going. And going.

I think people were very surprised as they didn't know anyone else who had fed that long. I often got, "but doesn't she eat everything?" and "she's HOW old?" But I didn't really care, I had started reading about breastfeeding by then and the more I read the longer I continued to feed.

When G was 18 months, I was pregnant and miscarried (nothing new to me, it was my fourth.) In hospital for a D&C, the nurses on the ward were fascinated with me, this woman feeding an18 month old. One nurse actually said that it affects fertility, and there I was already pregnant!

Anyhow, I was pregnant again three months later and I phoned La Leche league about what to do. I found them, and continue to find them, a huge support. And hugely knowledgable.

I now have two daughters and am tandem feeding reluctantly, cos somehow or other feeding G seems odd, but I continue cos she loves it and it's good for her and I hope and think it might control the sibling rivalry thing. It's a tough time for any child, so at least something is still hers.

I don't tell many that I feed both, hardly anybody in fact, which on writing makes me a bit sad, cos really it should be celebrated. G has been very good about her sister and loves her, I think our close relationship thru breastfeeding has definitely helped.

Breastfeeding: The Early Days
What's Not Normal...

For starters, let's talk about pain. Pain is not normal. Discomfort? Yes, initially that's normal. Pain that lasts a few seconds when your baby latches but then goes away? This can also be normal but should still be checked just in case. Pain that has you gritting your teeth as fiery daggers stab your breasts and shards of broken glass are sucked through your cracked, bleeding nipples? Definitely not normal.

This kind of pain means that something isn't right. Latch and positioning are two popular culprits, as are breast infection, blocked ducts, thrush or your baby's suck. Get the hospital lactation consultant to come and check both you and the baby out. Do not let anyone tell you that this is "Normal." If the latch and positioning are grand and there are no obvious causes of the pain (thrush, mastitis, vasospasms, etc...) check to see if your baby has a tongue tie. No matter what, do not "accept" this kind of pain as par for the course. Keep investigating until you find and solve the root of the problem. Contact your Local La Leche League, Cuidiu branch (Irish Childbirth Trust) or Breastfeeding Support Group for more information.

Constipation in the exclusively breastfed baby (never had anything other then breast milk, no water, formula, glucose syrup, medications, etc...) is not normal. In fact, it is so rare that there is hardly any literature on it at all. It is normal for breastfed babies to go days and days without a poo (or to poo several times a day for that matter!) but so long as the poo, when it eventually does arrive, is nice and runny, then you're baby is probably not constipated . If your exclusively breast fed baby starts doing

poos that are toothpaste consistency or harder though, take
them to your doctor to be checked out. This is not normal.

On the other hand, if your baby has received any substance
other then breast milk, constipation could rear it's ugly head, in
which case, see your doctor or lactation consultant for advice.

Colic. Contrary to popular belief, true colic in the breast fed
baby is not normal. There is almost always a reason for it.
Again, contact your doctor, lactation consultant or other certi-
fied, breastfeeding professional to help you get to the root of the
problem. Dr. Jack Newman has some great info on Colic and
the breastfed baby on his website.

Insufficient/No milk supply. While this can happen, it is very
rare and most definitely not normal. Most supply issues can
be solved or improved with help from an informed lactation
professional.

Jacquie's Story
I could ramble on about how tough I found the first few weeks
but I'm not going to because to be honest I think that life in the
first few weeks with a newborn is tough enough, whatever way
you decide to feed them.

Yes, we had oversupply and fast let-down, resulting in a windy
baby in the early weeks, but with time and the support of my
wonderful husband, my sister and a lactation consultant I got
through that and I'm so so glad we did.

Why? Because it is one thing me and our daughter share that
no one else gets with her (how selfish am I?!) Because my heart
still melts when she rolls off after a big feed with milk dribbling
down her chin, looks into my eyes and gives me a massive grin
before letting out a huge burp of satisfaction; because I get such
a kick when people say how alert/active/social she is and that
she's clearly thriving so keep doing what I'm doing! I grew her

inside me for 41 weeks and I'm still growing her now; because no matter how hectic life gets I have such a special excuse to sit and cuddle our gorgeous girl.

For me when I got pregnant there was never any question I would breastfeed and I think that is why I persisted, because to me it simply was the only way to feed our daughter r- there was no choice. I never went to LLL or cuidu meetings before Charlotte arrived, because it simply never occurred to me that we would have problems breastfeeding. And if we did it didn't matter - we would find a solution.

I always said before Charlotte arrived that it was weird to keep breastfeeding once your child got teeth, now that we've got to 24 weeks I can't imagine not breastfeeding Charlotte and fully intend to keep it up as long as either of us wants.

Real Mams Talk About:
Breastfeeding – The Early Days

The early days were tough. I'll be honest, I was totally clueless! I remember trying to get Aisling to latch on when I was in hospital and I thought I had it, she was sucking away for a good thirty minutes when the nurse arrived to see how I was getting on. Well, there was I with a big smile on my face, "yes she's flying, she's latched on and is feeding away!" The Nurse came forward to have a look. She broke the latch and there I was with a big, huge purple "love bite" right above my left nipple!!!! You can imagine how stupid I felt. I soon learnt what it really felt like when the baby latched correctly... On the nipple! I had expected it to be a lot easier. I honestly thought it would just happen with no pain, soreness, discomfort, anything but I soon learnt that it was a lot harder than that and that I needed to persist and I'd get there.

Eimear

Having had a general anesthetic for my c section meant that I missed Aoife being 'born' but my first memory of her is looking down at her latched onto me in the recovery room. It was such an amazing and surreal moment!

Nicola

No! The early days for me were awful. I think I used the words "barbaric" and "torturous" a lot and questioned exactly how it could be described as a "natural" experience. If it was such a "natural" thing to do, how come I didn't know how to do it?!? And I really didn't know how. I had the latch and positioning all wrong for five whole weeks before a lactation consultant helped me do it right. I hadn't a clue about the reality of demand-feeding a newborn baby (could she REALLY be hungry again? I just fed her an hour ago!) I asked the lovely ladies on the breastfeeding forum on rollercoaster though and was soon reassured on this count.

Adrienne

Brilliant, once the babies realized what I was doing! I loved every minute of it. Both of my children were naturals once they had been helped on the first time. With my daughter, I found it a little tougher as I was running around after my little boy! I had no problems health wise, apart from getting very tired, and my little girl was a very hungry baby and always wanted to be latched on!!

Christine, 29, Wicklow

They were exhausting. She was born with jaundice and the pressure was there to give her a bottle but I had good encouragement from one nice midwife. My milk came in on day two and her jaundice cleared up but I was faced with terrible nipple pain as I was unaware for a long time that I had her latched on wrong. I felt like crying. She was stuck to me 24/7 and I thought I would never get a break again.

Lucretia, 20, Dublin

With my first baby, the first few days were agony. I was not prepared for the pain. My milk took five days to come in and I had cracked and bleeding nipples. I used to do a silent scream whenever my son latched on. I used a lanolin based cream and forged on. By day five the pain had gone and there was plenty of milk. My son was nine pounds at birth and I was pressured by my husband on night three into giving him a bottle because my husband thought the baby was "starving." I felt awful and never again gave him another bottle. With my second baby (nine pounds ten ounces) there was less pain and the milk came in much faster. Both my babies were easily distracted during feeds but never lost weight, even after birth. Both of them were also fast feeders (ten to fifteen minutes) but I always produced a lot of milk so that helped.

Angela, 35, Dublin

I loved it from the very beginning, he took to it right away and I didn't have any difficulties which of course helps! Having said that, it was tiring and he fed every couple of hours but all I wanted was to cuddle my baby anyway so I really didn't mind.

Lisa, 32, Dublin

Eamonn stopped breathing shortly after he was born so he was put on machines to help him breathe for the three days. It was only when he was put into the incubator three days later that I was allowed to pick him up and feed him. I will never forget how excited I was when the nurses called me and told me he was looking to be fed. I ran down the stairs (as fast as you can run after a c-section!) to get to him. My mind was made up then that we were going to succeed with the breastfeeding no matter what. I wanted to help him anyway I could. It took a few days for him to learn to latch on but the midwives in the Special Care Unit were brilliant and gave me loads of help and support. By the time we left on day five, he was a pro.

Grainne, 34, Cork

It was really how I expected. I was sore, but I just kept watching videos online of babies latching, comparing that to what I was doing, and continuing on. I knew that if I could get past the early days it would get easier-- or else women wouldn't breast-feed for so long!

Candace, 24, Waterford

My first baby was in the special care unit for four or five days, so I had to express milk initially - not exactly the start I had imagined. It was really tough to get a good latch but one night, about day four we had a fantastic midwife who made it her mission to get us up and running properly by morning - and she did! I was also very engorged which was very painful and made it hard to get Hannah latched on. The first two weeks were much tougher than I expected but as everyone told me, it did get much easier and by about six weeks I would say that it was going well for us. On my second time around I had a c-section and although I was concerned this might make it more difficult for us, it was a doddle compared to the first time!

Muriel, 33, Dublin

Look at the baby - not the scale
by Jay Gordon, MD, FAAP, IBCLC
Dr. Gordon is the first male physician to sit and pass the the International Board of Lactation Certification Exam and has served on the Professional Advisory Board of La Leche League for twenty four years. This article has been reprinted here with his kind permission.

It sounds simple doesn't it? Yet I have seen so many moms whose babies have looked healthy, nursed well, met developmental milestones one right after the other and have lost all confidence in breastfeeding due to someone telling them that their baby's weight was not on the charts. This someone was looking at the scale and charts, rather than the baby.

In the first 24 to 72 hours after birth babies tend to lose about 3-10% of their birth weight and then regain that weight over the next 2 to 3 weeks. If a mother receives lots of IV fluids during labor, the baby could be born "heavier" because of the increased water. The somewhat higher weight could be measured if a baby were weighed right before it peed for the first time. The difference of this extra fluid retention might only be a few ounces, but some parents are told to be concerned when, at their baby's two week checkup, the baby is a few ounces under birth weight.

Another common problem at early checkups is a baby that is not gaining what the practitioner considers to be "normal weight gain." There is not general agreement on normal weight gain and the range in texts are from 4 to 8 ounces a week. Some babies are genetically destined to be a lot smaller or larger than others. As I mentioned in the first paragraph: Easy concept, isn't it?

If you have been told that weight gain is not acceptable, look hard at this list of questions:

* Is your baby eager to nurse?
* Is your baby peeing and pooping well?
* Is your baby's urine either clear or very pale yellow?
* Are your baby's eyes bright and alert?
* Is your baby's skin a healthy color and texture?
* Is your baby moving its arms and legs vigorously?
* Are baby's nails growing?
* Is your baby meeting developmental milestones?
* Is your baby's overall disposition happy and playful?
* Yes, your baby sleeps a lot, but when your baby is awake does he have periods of being very alert?

If you have answered yes to the above questions, you may want to progress on to two important questions which the "charts" seem to ignore.

* How tall is mom?
* How tall is dad?

If someone were to ask you what weight a 33 year old man should be, you would laugh. The range of possibilities varies according to height, bone structure, ethnicity and many other factors. Yet babies are expected to fit onto charts distributed throughout the country with no regard to genetics, feeding choice or almost anything else.

There can be nursing problems that can cause slow weight gain; an inadequate "latch-on" is probably the only common breastfeeding problem in the first weeks. This is an easily remedied problem with the right help. In the best of circumstances, breastfeeding should be assessed within the first day or two after birth by a skilled lactation expert. Good hospitals have these LC's and IBCLC's on staff and, if not, please line up a consultation within the first 12 hours of life. Your pediatrician can help you with this. If not, call La Leche League and ask them whom they recommend in your area. This is a crucial step in becoming a parent and must not be skipped.

If there are nursing problems, the first answer should never be supplementation but must be to find the best advice and help available. Find quality help in person if possible and on line if needed. There is nothing better than having an experienced breastfeeding expert watch you and your baby and give you the help and encouragement and support you need and deserve. Too many mothers and babies lose the breastfeeding experience and the lifesaving and illness preventing benefits because we doctors are trained to look harder at the scale than we are at the baby.

A few notable examples:

* Baby, birth weight: 9 lbs. 12 oz.
Weight 36 hours after delivery: 9 lbs. 2 oz.

I have seen mothers encouraged to supplement because "they have no milk, the baby is hungry and losing weight." The baby looks good and is nursing every 1 to 3 hours and mom's nipples are not getting sore. There is no need to do anything but nurse often and wait another day or two for the milk to come in. A thirsty baby nurses strongly and is in no danger. A baby given water or formula might not nurse so strongly and mom's confidence (and milk supply) will suffer for it. This mom only needs the support of an expert who can be sure that she knows how to latch her baby on to the breast.

* Same baby, two week checkup: 9 lbs. 6 oz

Forgetting that this represents a 4 oz. weight gain from the 36 hour weight, some docs might recommend supplementation. Again, watch breastfeeding and if everything is going well, don't worry. A dry, jaundiced baby with darker yellow urine is a different case and needs more help with nursing. This baby still should not get formula. Make sure mom is drinking enough water, nursing often without a set schedule (every 1 to 3 hours) and make very sure that she gets help latching her baby on, especially if she has sore nipples.

* Same baby, six month checkup: 15 lbs.

Lactation consultation had been successful in the early weeks thanks to mom having found a supportive, smart doctor and being determined to succeed at feeding her baby the best. This big baby (9 lbs. 12 oz. at birth, remember?) had weighed 13 pounds at her four month visit and now weighs 15 pounds. The doctor is paying attention and sees that Mom is 5' 3" and Dad is 5' 9" and slender. He looks at the charts second and the baby first and isn't concerned about the baby dropping from a very high percentile at birth to a lower one and then to a lower one still.

I think I'll conclude this scenario with this happy ending.

In summary, babies who are nursing, peeing clear urine and wetting diapers well in the first weeks of life are almost always all right. I cannot recall seeing a baby for whom slow weight gain in the first 2 to 6 weeks was the only sign of a problem.

Older babies, 2 to 12 months of age, grow at varying rates. Weight gain should not be used as a major criterion of good health. Developmental milestones and interaction with parents and others are more important. Do not be persuaded to supplement a baby who is doing well. Get help with breastfeeding and use other things besides weight to guide you.

Real Mams Talk About:
Breastfeeding Support

I was lucky that my mom and dad were with me for the first three weeks and that I also had my husband's support. They just kept encouraging me and took control of everything else that needed to be done, so I could focus solely on getting the hang of breastfeeding and relaxing. I turned towards the internet a lot as well to interact with other new breastfeeding moms. I looked forward to nap times when I could go online and share with these women how my day was going. It was a great sounding board for me. I eventually joined a mom and baby group run by a lactation consultant and felt empowered by being around other women who had the same goals in mind.

Some of my husband's family were not as supportive, especially once we were out of the newborn stage. They tried to rattle off their beliefs about what was right in terms of raising children as they were all much older than me and most of them believed that there was absolutely no difference between bottle and breast which made me feel that all my hard work for my little girl was really underestimated.

They did not hold back their opinions that I should stop breastfeeding once my daughter was more than a few months old. I received looks (from the women, not the men) when I would nurse at the family home when my daughter was over a year, as if they were creeped out by the whole thing. It made me feel very insecure and saddened. Although my husband was very supportive, it was hard for him to explain the breastfeeding benefits to his family.

Erin, 31, Cork

My husband's support was one of the main factors in my succeeding. He was unwavering, never questioned how often Ella fed, how much she was getting, he was brilliant. My PHN was great too, but I always got the impression that she didn't see many breastfeeding mums because she was so enthused to see us feeding.

In the hospital I got help, but not of the helpful kind. Quite frankly I felt like I was annoying the nurses, one even wrote a snide , "Mother needs constant help with feeding," in my notes. Not so helpful. And I was never offered a Lactation Consultant (perhaps because it was the weekend? who knows!) Family and friends were all supportive but as Ella has grown, I have been getting vibes that they are embarrassed by her feeding and think I'm a little eccentric to be feeding so long!

Kate, 31, Galway

On my first baby, I had to express for the first couple of weeks as William was seven weeks premature. I got loads of support from the nurses in the special baby care unit, which was really appreciated as William kept falling asleep at the breast. I was surprised though, and I'm still very upset that the pediatrician prescribed one bottle of formula milk plus vitamins and iron for him per day. I thought that breast was best - especially for premature babies - but everyone I asked just said, "Sure it won't do him any harm and it will give you a break."

It made his bottom bleed and they spent a couple of days in the hospital investigating the bleeding. It eventually cleared up at four months when I felt confident enough to go against medical opinion and take him off the formula.

My mother in law thought I should give up (breastfeeding) at six months, my family thought I should give up at one year, the doctor thought I should give up when I got pregnant. I eventually gave up at three months pregnant as I was sore and tired. William was fourteen months old. I am still feeding Peter (my second) at twenty months (much to the family's disgust.)

Catherine

Aisling was born in hospital by way of c-section (she was breech.) Support, to be honest, wasn't great. On our first night , the nurse on duty told me she'd take Aisling from me and bring her to the nursery to give me a break. I politely declined, there was no way I was letting her out of my sight and anyway, I really wanted to give the feeding a go. The nurse turned and said, "Oh sure, you can give her a bottle tonight! It really isn't going to do her any harm!" That's the level of support I got.

During my four day stay, I can honestly say that I received no "decent" support. In fact, I ended up ringing my sister who had breastfed her three children to answer any questions I had and have continued to do so to this day. On leaving the hospital, I got the standard booklet that's handed to everyone which did have a number for the lactation consultant which I've never used.

Eimear, Cork

My mother in law was against it because she failed on her first and never tried again. She said it would wear me out and couldn't believe I wanted to try breastfeeding again on baby two. I am still feeding baby two once a day and she is almost three now. My mother in law has grown used to it and actually changed her negative ideas about breastfeeding into positive ones!

The support from health professionals however is unchanged. They still know very little about breastfeeding, I feel like I'm the expert. Only positive was my GP, quite an old man delighted to hear that I was still feeding my two year old when pregnant with number three.

Mam of three, 28

I had great support from my mother and my partner but everyone else was like, "Are you sure she's getting enough?" and "Sure, isn't a bottle as good as breast milk these days?" I still get good support from my mother and partner but everyone else thinks I should have stopped by now. They seem to think that breastfeeding an older child is wrong and that I'm trying to be some kind of martyr.

Lucretia, 20, Dublin

I got great support from Cúidiu, La Leche League, and Irish internet forums. Family and Friends were a bit cautious of it. Whenever I had a problem or a sore breast, I was told by my family, "You've done enough. It's okay that you have to stop now." No one ever asked did I want to stop... Which I didn't!

Alanna, 25, Cork

There was a great German mid-wife in the hospital, but to be honest, I needed no help. I had done a breastfeeding class three weeks before my daughter was born thus I knew it might be difficult, so I had a mate lined up to help me if I go into trouble. I thought she was a good resource as she had not managed to feed her first but managed really well on her second. So I thought she would be objective. But in the end my German mid-wife told my husband that it was like she was dealing with a 3rd or 4th time mum and she just left me happily to it all. It was great.

The public health nurse was a joke. Bronagh had put on 11oz in a week – double the supposed target. My mid-wife still suggested I should express to see if I had "enough supply"????? I mean hello - 11oz. If she knew anything at all about breastfeeding (which her comment showed she was and is completely under qualified and under educated to be helping any new mother!) she would have known that the amount you get from expressing and actual baby feeding can be completely different.

Some friends actually challenge me openly now that I have chosen to extend feed. I have never said now why did you feed your child formula – do you know what it does etc? But they now feel that they can challenge my decision to extend feed. And I know they think I am a freak. Someday soon I will point out to them that I am very happy with my decision and I have never asked them why they never even bothered to feed a new born never mind a child over a year – I respected their decision, why can't they accept mine? I have also had to have a little bit of a battle with my husband. He feels a lot the science behind extended feeding has actually been made up by the breastfeeding "Nazi's." But he still has left me to it.

Cita, 33, Kildare

The only support I had in the early days of breastfeeding were various online forums. I went to my first La Leche League meeting when my daughter was five months old and it was the best thing I ever did. Suddenly, I wasn't an oddball and I met a lot of strong women. I met my best friend there and am even a La Leche League leader applicant now.

Candace, 24, Waterford

Dad, here's how to support breastfeeding...
(A great big thank you to Friends of Breastfeeding who were kind enough to provide this article from their outstanding breastfeeding information pack.)

Your support is essential to helping your partner to breastfeed your baby. Yes, breastfeeding is something that happens between a mother and child but it can take time for both to learn the skill and while they do, it is important that they receive support and care. A recent study in Sligo (First Time Father's

Experience of Breast Feeding, Liz Martin, Health Promotion Officer at the HSE) revealed that the decision to breastfeed was influenced strongly and positively by the father.

What can you do for your partner?

Read and learn about the benefits of breastfeeding.

Help your partner and child to feel comfortable while feeding – offer cushions, bring her a drink and a healthy snack.

Help your partner check your baby's positioning and latch.

Prepare meals and take care of housework, do the shopping.

Encourage your partner to accept as much help as possible.

Talk to your partner and express your feelings.

Encourage, reassure and listen to your partner when she is tired or finding things difficult.

Explain to family members and friends about the importance of a creating a supportive environment while breastfeeding is established. Protect her from unhelpful comments and opinions.

What can you do for your baby?

Firstly, anything you do to support your partner will be good for your baby! Feeding is only one thing that a baby needs but there are many other ways to help care for your child.

Share skin-to-skin time with your baby - lay your child on your bare chest, holding him, stroking him, let him nap there.

Bath your baby.

Take your baby for walks in the pram, or carry your baby in a sling.

Massage your baby.

Talk to your baby. Read and sing to your baby.

Change your baby's nappy.

Bring your baby to your partner for feeds.

Settle your baby after feeds, wind your baby, and soothe your baby.

Remember:

Breastfeeding works on supply and demand. Newborn babies especially will feed frequently – the more they feed, the more milk will be made. Your partner will need extra support at these times.

Keeping mum and baby together at night will help feeding on demand.

If your baby is having wet and dry nappies and gaining weight normally, you can be reassured that they are getting enough milk.

Breastfeeding should be well established before introducing any sort of fluids from a bottle

since the type of sucking required to breastfeed is different to that required to feed from a bottle.

Your partner might like to meet with other breastfeeding mums. Your Public Health Nurse will know about local breastfeeding groups (Cuidiú or LLL) or check out www. friendsofbreastfeeding.ie

Feeding in Public: Kate's story

The first time I ever fed in public was when Olivia was four weeks old. My mother, grandmother, husband and I were out for lunch at Avoca. I felt very conspicuous but my mother assured me that no one was looking. We managed just fine although I know I was going red and trying not to meet anyone's gaze! It was difficult because sometimes if we weren't getting a good latch Olivia would come off the breast and I would feel nervous that she would expose me.

I remember eating dinner in a Thai restaurant with six friends. I had to leave the table to feed her in the disabled toilet standing up! I just didn't have the confidence to feed her at the table because she made such a fuss that people were looking over at us and giving us dirty looks. I pretty much got over my fear about feeding her in public when I had to sit next to an elderly man on a bench in the middle of a shopping centre in Newry! I think a lot of times people don't actually realize what you are doing. I haven't had any real negative reactions except for some people staring.

Every time I see another nursing mother in public my heart always does a little flip. I feel a bit more confident and a sense of kinship with her! I am happy to say that I have breastfed on a beach, in a car, on a plane, in numerous restaurants, on a boat, in front of the men in my family... everywhere, and I don't feel any shame about it.

Real Mam's Talk about...
Feeding in Public

I wasn't very confident in the early days about breastfeeding in public. Our first solo outing saw me order a Panini and cappuccino - only to have my son wake up as soon as I had taken my first bite. He was wet and proceeded to roar so I left my untouched lunch there and went to change him in the tiny, completely unsuitable baby change cubicle. I spent more time in there than I did at the table. If I remember correctly, it was about about thirty minutes as, true to form, he wanted a feed as well. I fed him standing up as there was nowhere to sit down. It was a horrible experience that did nothing for my confidence.

Today, however, I would feed on the altar at noon mass on a Sunday if the situation arose. Indeed, I have fed in the church at my nephews communion. I've also "done it" in a swimming pool, at the zoo, standing up at the bottom of the escalator in Dundrum, on a bench in a park, on a bench in the middle of many shopping centers, in my parents house, in my in-laws, in the bank, in work, my doctors waiting room, on the banks of a canal. I've come a long way!

Gwen, Kildare

It took me a good while to work up the confidence to feed out-side of home. I felt shy and uncomfortable about latching her on in public- that fumbling movement of me unhooking the bra strap and lifting my top, but I'm an expert by now. I don't even bother unhooking the bra, just hoik the whole lot up in the one go and off she goes. I can now feed anywhere, anytime. I can even feed standing up. It's great! So far I have never received any sort of reaction, neither positive nor negative. I think people mostly don't see what they don't expect to see.

Adrienne

Once William got to a year, I felt more self conscious. But this didn't happen with Peter until he reached about fifteen months. I was in playgroup feeding him as discreetly as I could and the Dutch woman next to me said, "I'm still feeding my daughter as well." Her daughter was two and a half years and since then, I don't care.

Catherine, 37, Dublin

To my own surprise feeding in public never fazed me. Due to the section I didn't go out for about two months by which time I was very confident feeding. I feed in public a lot and have never had any comments, negative or positive. I am a little more self-conscious feeding a toddler but I still do it and still have had no comments.

Shirley, 36

Tandem Toddlers: Jen's Story
(kindly borrowed with permission from the author)
When I was pregnant with my first I hoped to feed her until she was six months; never did it cross my mind that 3 years down the line I'd not only still be feeding her but also feeding her little sister My girls are 17 months and 32 months and both nurse a couple of times a day.

We've come a long way since our nervous beginnings; from the initial few days of figuring out what goes where and the first time nursing in public. On that first outing my mum came with me. I had dressed carefully, taking advice from an online breastfeeding forum to wear a layer I could pull down and a layer I could pull up, thus enabling tiny to latch on while remaining discreet. After a bit of fumbling about and my mums reassurance that all flesh was contained I sat back and nursed my little one.

Over the following weeks I got braver and stopped fretting about discretion. I soon realized that it made more sense to wear something that could be pulled up and down quickly as opposed to a discreet but intricate system. Soon we were nursing in slings, while shopping, while out walking, there was nowhere that us two experts could not nurse.

When my daughter was six months we began to gently introduce solids through the baby led weaning approach and a few weeks after that we discovered I was pregnant again so we then went through the ups and downs of pregnant nursing. She weaned at 13 ½ months when my milk dried up, I was almost 8 months pregnant, but a year later she decided that she wanted to nurse again. So just like that, I was tandem feeding toddlers.

Toddler nursing and in particular toddler tandem nursing is a long way from the gentle baby days where my little darling would suckle quietly as I chatted to friends. No longer is nursing time signaled by a little one nuzzling in her sling, gently mewling for a feed, now it's loud and proud toddlers in the seat of the shopping trolley screaming 'BOOBIE NOW.'

When my girls were infants I'd feed them on demand, anytime anywhere,now I often try to hold them off with a cup of water or a sandwich until it's a little more convenient for me.

Gone is the cradle hold, the football hold and the gentle positioning techniques. The minute I take my top off to get dressed or have a shower, tiny greedy eyes light up and I'll generally just lean over or kneel and they'll stand there, arms hugging me, feeding. If I sit on the couch I'm in danger of being clambered on, my top wrenched up and a little one snuggling in for a feed. They feed their dolls, they get me to feed their dolls. My 2 ½ year old will tell you proudly,'I have nipple boobs now but when I a big woman I have big boobies and feed my baby that comes out my 'gina.' Oh yes, they're growing up fast.

I've recently had to have a little chat with my girls to explain to them that mummy's boobies are 'private' and when we're visiting people they either take turns feeding or we go somewhere 'private' where they can both feed together. Feeding time is not so much about feeding anymore as it is a family activity. To be honest it's gotten to be a bit of a production. Like anything else we do there is a lot of giggling, jostling, chatting, messing and general toddlers. This is all well and good but I've moved a little out of my comfort zone when I'm trying to have a conversation with another adult with my top up around my ears and two nutters wrestling over my boobs. I jokingly called it 'boobiefest' one day and it caught on.

'Mummy, I want a boobiefest NOW.'

'In a minute love, when I've finished cleaning up the little poo pile your sister left behind the couch.'

Did I mention I have to hum 'neeee, neeeee' while feeding? It started a few weeks ago when my oldest was complaining that her little sister had emptied 'her' boob. I pretended to fill it up while making the aforementioned 'neee' sound. Bad mistake. Himself thinks it's hilarious and keeps suggesting to the girls that I ought to make a 'bing' noise when it's full. Pity I can't reach to kick him when the two savages are nursing.

Everything about our nursing relationship feels right to me and totally normal. I'm not sure how long this wonderful part of our relationship will continue but we'll be at it as long as they like. We may be heading towards the outer reaches of parenting normality in this country but that's society's issue. My family are very happy, thank you very much.

Real Mams Talk About:
"Extended" Breastfeeding

My older daughter Hannah was exclusively breastfed until she was five and a half months old then gradually weaned to formula by the time she was seven months. I think in retrospect, the main reasons I weaned her at this point were because:

1. I'd told everyone I'd wean her at about six months.
2. I didn't really know anyone who'd continued much beyond six months.
3. I was feeling drained as she'd started waking again at night.

This time around with my younger girl, Kirsten, I'm still breast-feeding along with starting solids.

What I've only recently fully appreciated is that the six month mark is tough going because you're producing the maximum amount of milk at this point. It's right before the solids start kicking in and they often start waking more at night again.

From now on in it should get easier all the time in contrast to the constant growth spurts of the first six months. She has already dropped down from six or seven feeds a day to four feeds after only six weeks on solids so I'm finding it much easier again.

Also, this time around I don't feel like people really care what I do. They know I'm breastfeeding her. Last time, I felt like I was constantly reporting on progress, weight gain, etc... to first time grandparents and the like.

The other thing which is different for me this time is that although I knew the theory about the health benefits of breastfeeding with Hannah, I didn't fully appreciate the fact she'd never been sick until within a month of stopping breastfeeding, she was at the doctor three times with a bad skin rash and a horrendous bout of diarrhea which took two weeks to clear up.

Muriel, 33, Dublin

I know that if I breastfeed Colum over the year, I will have to either hide it from, or at the very least, definitely not mention it to my family as I believe they will think it's disgusting. I can't imagine feeding my two year old. Even the thought of it now makes me feel uncomfortable but I might feel differently when Colum reaches that age. As far as improving the public perception, haven't a clue. Only if things become the norm do people begin to accept it. Imagine asking a mother in the 60's or 70's how she would feel if her daughter moved in with her boyfriend before marriage - now it's seen as unusual, even weird if a couple don't live together before they are married.

Grainne, 34, Cork

I don't believe there is a cut-off point. For me my personal cut-off is very mobile, it always seems to be about three months older than Iz is at any given time. At the moment I am saying two, but who knows? Until Iz was one, I was very proud of the fact that I was breastfeeding and I enjoyed feeding her in public and speaking to people about it. Since she has started walking,

I have found myself talking about it less and less. I don't hide it, but I wouldn't mention it unless someone asked. I just don't know how they'll react. I sometimes feel bad about this because I believe the only way to improve public perception is to talk about it.

Shirley, 36, Dublin

As long as my daughter is hungry she will be fed regardless of where we are. But I have started to get those remarks from family members, "Oh, you have done the six months, sure can't you stop now?" I don't know where this "six months" came from. I plan to feed until she is two. This scares some of my family members. They think it's disgusting. It's because they are so badly educated about breastfeeding. One of my relatives believed that you dried up at six months. I think that there needs to be more restrictions on formula ads. A lot of this is generated by the "follow on milk after six months." It makes mothers believe that they aren't enough for their baby anymore.

Lucretia, 20, Dublin

I wouldn't argue with breastfeeding toddlers, but my gut feeling has always been that for me, I don't want to argue with a child who can talk about whether or not it's time for a feed in the middle of Tesco. Also, I wonder about independence, and separation from the mother in a healthy way? I'm not sure. I'm certainly going to feed my son longer than I did my daughter. Having read a lot more, it feels different... why stop giving him this miracle protection while it's available?

Jo, 32, Wicklow

To whom it may concern:
I know you're surprised. You think I've gone all hippy. But look at my most gorgeous children! They are happy, healthy and secure. And I'm so crazy about them.

Yes. She's three years old. Why am I feeding her? Well. I like to. She likes to. I feel close to her and she feels secure. She loves it. She says it's nicer than Kit-kats - I've asked her.

There are health benefits you know. She hasn't needed antibiotics to date. She has a very healthy appetite. Yes, of course, none of us were breastfed and we're okay, but is that a good measure? Are we okay? People get over the most awful of times, but these awful times leave their mark. So that's not a measure.

There's more than enough evidence to show this is good for my children. Anyhoo, it seems to me that since the world stopped breastfeeding, there's a lot more violence, teenage problems, crime, adults needing psychotherapy, etc... You know this "teenage" thing only started in the 60's. Coincidence?

You say I'm doing it for myself? Like an addiction? Hmmm... would you like to try and breastfeed either of my girls? See what I mean? You can't force a child to breastfeed. Don't mean to be rude, but that's nonsense. Did you know that up to recent times, the average age of weaning was 4 years?

I can't understand your difficulty with my doing something that's so patently good and wholesome for everyone. Is it the exposed boobs bit? I've been feeding for three years, have you ever seen much? Even if you have, which I doubt, what's the problem? Its a boob. Big deal. You see them everyday, somewhere. Here, have a read of chapters one and two in this book I have here. And then tell me more of the reasons you think I should stop.

You say I'm tied? What do you do, where do you go that's so untied? They're small children, I'm not leaving them, breastfed or not, and we (DH and I) have no desire to leave them, for a weekend away or whatever. So you can call it tied. I call it happy.

You might think and say I'm nuts, but really, I don't care, this is how it's meant to be, and it suits all of us in our home. It makes us all happy.

So, how are things with you? Hope you're all well.

Sincerely,
Mairead

Overcoming Challenges: Emma's Story

All throughout my pregnancy on my daughter Ailís, I had pretty much decided that I was going to give breastfeeding a go. My husband and I had both been breastfed for some bit and in both our families nearly everyone had breastfed at least a while. I assumed that because breastfeeding was the most natural and normal way for a baby to be fed, that it was going to be easy, so much so that I didn't bother buying a tin of formula to have just in case, as advised at the anti-natal class . Unfortunately it turned out to be a bit more difficult than I had expected.

At 38 weeks + 3days my waters broke at home and 36 hours later, after 18 hours of active labour, our darling daughter arrived by emergency c-section weighing 9lbs 1 oz. I was in shock. Following my section I was brought to recovery and once I was settled the very kind nurse and midwife helped me to get my daughter latched on. It took a couple of goes because I could hardly move, but we eventually got her latched on. It was an amazing if slightly weird feeling, but not in a bad way.

The first few days in hospital were very tough. I found it very hard to move, my blood pressure was all over the place, I couldn't sleep and every time I went to feed my little woman I was in agony. Every single midwife who saw me feeding said there was nothing wrong with the latch so they didn't know why I was in pain. I was told that it was normal and that it would just pass. One of the best tips I got to help heal cracked nipples was to rub a little bit of your milk into your nipple when you'd finished feeding and to leave it air dry.

By day three she'd had a couple of top ups of formula and I was ready to give up. I really didn't think I could go on but I also didn't want to give up that early as I felt that I had already failed her by not having delivered her naturally and I wasn't going to fail her again.

That night she fed away but was still fussing after about twenty to thirty minutes of being on the boob. In floods of tears I rang the bell and within minutes there was a lovely midwife called Mary standing at the end of my bed, asking was I alright. I told here that I had just fed Ailís but she still seemed hungry and could she please top her up. She checked Ailís over and agreed that yes she was probably was hungry as her lips were dry and cracked. So she sat at the end of my bed and gave Ailís some formula from a syringe, she was the only one of the midwives to do this the rest had just used bottles.

We started chatting and she promised to help me get the breast-feeding sorted if that's what I really wanted to do. I told her it was. The rest of that night was brilliant. Mary took Ailís to the nursery so I could get some rest and would bring her back for a feed when she woke up. At around 1:00 am Mary arrived back with Ailís and I started to get out of the bed to go sit on the chair to feed her. Mary told me to stay where I was that I could feed lying down. Feed lying down and doze while baby sleeps, this is the first I heard of it.

So I lay down got all comfy and Mary helped me to latch Ailís on and she fed and she really fed! I could feel my milk coming in and hear the sound of it as it hit her empty tummy and there was never such a sweeter sound to be heard. It was amazing still painful, but absolutely amazing. To this day I still love the sound of milk hitting a new baby's empty tummy. She fed for over twenty five minutes during which time we both dozed. After that she stayed with me and two days later we were sent home.

The next few weeks flew by in a blur, as it does for everyone with a new baby. My only problem was that I used to get afraid every time she got hungry as I knew the pain that awaited me. Some days were worse than others. There were a couple of nights where my husband would have to get me some pain killers as I was feeding her and others where he would literally have to push her face to my boob as I just couldn't bring myself to let her latch on. Some days I gave in and gave her a bottle sometimes of formula and others of expressed milk and I used to cry every time I put a bottle into her mouth. I felt like such a mean useless Mammy for not even being able to feed her.

At this stage both our families were telling me to just give up that I had done my best, that there was no need to torture myself, yet I couldn't bring myself to do it. I just couldn't. At one stage when Ailís was about seven or eight weeks old my Mam said to me "Emma just piss or get off the pot, one or the other your either breastfeeding or you're not but you need to decide". So I did. That weekend there was a La Leche coffee morning in Midleton for National Breastfeeding week so I went along in the hopes that I might get some help. Why oh why did I not get in touch with them sooner???

Ailís and I sat at a table by ourselves as I didn't know anyone there, then J came over and we got chatting. It turns out she was one of the Counsellors from La Leche in the city and she had come up to say hi to everyone. She was a star. She sat with me for the whole morning and we chatted and she watched as I fed Ailís. Like the midwives in the hospital she could see nothing wrong with our latch, Ailís was drinking away no problems and most importantly she was thriving. And then she looked again and ever so gently she just slightly rotated Ailís hip and bum into my hand more. It was a movement of no more than a fraction of an inch but instantly the pain stopped! Oh my God how good that felt! It turns out that because she was such a big baby and a wriggler that I had difficulty in keeping her whole body turned into me and that was why it hurt so much. After that I was incredibly conscious of how I held her when feeding and within a few days it became second nature to me.

I enjoyed every minute of feeding her from then on. I now looked forward to sitting down and nursing her instead of dreading it. It was so incredibly relaxing and I remember describing it to once to my Mam as being in a state of nirvana, it was just so calming and relaxing for both of us. Not only did I enjoy our special chill out time together but I used to get such a wonderful feeling of empowerment knowing that it was my milk that was sustaining her and letting her thrive. Very few people could believe that a breastfed baby could sleep the night through from ten weeks and have dropped to four feeds a day by four months and still continue to thrive without some other source of nourishment, but she did.

We continued to enjoy our breastfeeding experience together until Ailís was a year and two weeks old. I was six months pregnant on baby number two and I feel that her weaning was pretty much a mutual agreement. By that stage she was down to one feed a day, having dropped most of the others herself, and I was getting sick of having to chase her around the house and hold her down to feed her before bed. So one night I'd had enough and gave her a cup of warm milk and honey instead of the boob, just to see how she would react. She guzzled the lot and never once looked for the boob. I was sorry that our breastfeeding journey together had ended but I was also incredibly proud of myself as never in a million years did I think that I would get to the one year mark never mind feed whilst pregnant with another baby.

What was the Most Challenging Aspect of Breastfeeding for You?

The biggest challenge to me is peoples attitudes, from medical staff to friends and family. I was so disappointed with the support, or lack of, that I received after having Aisling. To be honest I can see why people don't decide to breastfeed, why would you when you are encouraged to give a bottle! Truth be told without the support of my family I don't know how successful I would have been. Overcoming peoples attitudes is difficult but being strong and remaining positive about breastfeeding has helped me overcome it, I can see the benefits of breastfeeding Aisling and strongly believe in breastfeeding which helps when you come up against those doubting Thomas' out there!

Eimear, Cork

Oh dear. I found all of it a challenge at the start. I took it as such a shock to the system. I didn't understand the reality of demand feeding and just how demanding it can be for the first two weeks. I felt isolated in having nobody close to me to ask for help or advice in the early days. I felt tortured with the pain, pain, pain of doing it all wrong it those early weeks! In later weeks I lacked confidence and shyness at feeding in public but this was gradually overcome, the more I did it.

I researched every morsel of information I could get a hold of regarding breastfeeding, on the internet. I could only feed comfortably lying down in the early weeks, which scuppered any hopes I had of ever leaving the house with my new baby. At five weeks I contacted a lactation consultant, who came to my house and helped me position my daughter in the cross cradle hold. My own feeble attempts at the cradle hold left me with traumatized nipples resulting in nipple blanching which a treatment of osteopathy finally sorted out at ten weeks. In that meantime there was also a number of occurrences of blocked ducts, which I am adept at treating myself now.

Adrienne

Feeling touched out, for sure. It's hard because sometimes you want your body to yourself. It's hard when your partner is waiting his turn for your boobs and when the time comes you want them for yourself!

Candace, 24, Waterford

There were several challenging aspects. One huge one is not being able to give baby to someone else to feed for a change. My husband totally gave over all feeding responsibilities to me and this included nappy changes etc... because I felt it was pointless to wake him up to change the nappies when I was already up and he had to go to work. He used to follow me around the house though and say to me, "He needs to be fed!" If the child whimpered for a second, my husband would call me and say he needed to be fed. Everything was down to he needs to be fed.

I found the lack of support to be a little overwhelming. If I had a euro for the amount of times people said, would you not just give him a bottle, I'd be a rich lady now. The medical profession weren't much better. I went to my GP with what I pretty much knew to be thrush on my nipples and he practically laughed me out of the surgery and told me to keep feeding and come back to him if it didn't get better. I suffered with horrible pain for a month until I eventually rang the hospital when I could hardly lift my baby or push the pram and they told me to come in and it was diagnosed and I got treatment. I did feel very let down.

The breastfeeding support group in my area consisted of people queuing up to have the baby weighed and that was it. I felt very much alone and if I had any complaints, people would look at me and say, well if you gave up breastfeeding he'll sleep through the night and pretty much put every problem down to breastfeeding so I therefore got very little sympathy if things weren't going well. I did find that the ladies on rollercoaster were a godsend and were inspirational and kept me going when I had very low moments. I wouldn't have lasted as long as I did without them.

Joanna, 38, Dublin

Getting the babies to take long feeds as neither really did; also they often detached and had to latch on again. I was told by the lactation consultant that it was because of an over abundant supply of milk startling them. But we managed in the end, I am glad I persevered.

Angela, 35, Dublin

The first few weeks of feeding my oldest baby. I was very innocent about the whole thing and I didn't understand the whole concept of feeding on demand and him sitting under me in the evenings. The sore nipples got to me, but it wasn't bad enough to put me off and it went away after nine or ten days. None of my three children have ever taken to bottles. so that is a very big negative for me. I am very restricted. So my second baby (girl) I put her on bottles at eight weeks cos she was refusing them and I regretted it ever since. I really wish I had fed her for longer. So what if she didn't take bottles? I wasn't really going anywhere. So now on my third baby, I'm feeding away six months later with no intention of giving up for a while yet.

Meadbh

I think maybe the lack of support, or the lack of normality about it all. Of course the tiredness, but motherhood IS tiring, and we shouldn't be led to believe otherwise.

Mairead

Real Mams Talk about:
Breastfeeding Advice to New Mams...

One of my main concerns before I breastfed was how self-conscious I'd be and that I'd never be able to breastfeed in front of anyone. When it actually happened I really didn't care - faced with a crying baby you've got to feed, it just becomes irrelevant. Also remember it does get so much easier - it is really tough going for the first six weeks or so, but gets easier all the time after that.

Muriel, 33, Dublin

Try try try. I was unsure whether to resume trying after leaving the hospital when my milk 'came in'. I was sat on the bed after having a shower and bottle feeding my little girl when I was leaking milk all over her. It was so ironic I burst into tears. It is a brilliant start to a baby's life and if you aren't too sure, you can't break the baby by trying. If it doesn't suit you or the baby, well at least you gave it a shot. Even combined feeding is highly satisfying.

Sarah, 28, Cork

My main piece of advice is DON'T GIVE UP when things are tough at the start, I promise you it does get easier. There were times (engorgement and cracked nipple) when I was ready to throw the towel in but I persisted and I am so glad I did. Also take advice from family members and friends who have breastfed they were a life saver to me, be proud that you breastfeed and don't let people put you off by being negative and making you feel you are doing something wrong. You are not! And if you are unsure my advice is log onto rollercoaster or a similar website and go to the breastfeeding thread, have a read through and post a question, the support you get from these sites is great and you know its honest as those postings are people going through same as you.

Eimear, Cork

Realizing that we as mothers are made to nourish or babies physically and emotionally is very empowering and I personally feel honored to have that privilege. I know that it can be challenging at times but can only say that it is worth it in gold. Few things are insurmountable and I wouldn't change a moment of those challenges for they make me value the wonderful nursing relationship I have with my now eighteen month old daughter all the more. There's so much more to it than milk!

Kara

Get a good book on breastfeeding and read it cover to cover. Anything by Jack Newman is recommended as is his website. Ina May's Guide to Breastfeeding is another wonderful source of information and support. Websites like Kellymom.com are filled to the brim with great breastfeeding advice and the breast-feeding boards on Irish parenting sites like rollercoaster.ie and magicmum.ie are invaluable. Look up your local breastfeeding group and start going to meetings while pregnant. This will give you a number of benefits.

Firstly, you will get to see loads of breastfeeding mothers and babies doing their thing in all different ways. Secondly, you will get to hear their experiences and know that more then likely, You can do this too. You will also hear about common problems in the early days and ways of rectifying them. Thirdly, you will meet other breastfeeding mums who will help form your support network when your baby is born and you begin nursing. They are great people to call when you need advice or just a shoulder to lean on. Oh! And there's usually tea and biscuits as well :)

J, 31, Wexford

Breastfeeding will be the most wonderful experience of your life. The most wonderful. How can you miss this experience? You've grown your baby very well for nine months, but there's a lot more growing to do and your little one needs breast milk to finish this growing properly. And she needs you for this.

She won't get sick so often, she's likely to have better teeth, she'll have a higher IQ, she'll have lovely skin, she'll be a confident happy adult, she'll have a healthier immune system forever and a hundred more reasons you'll find anywhere. If you're only playing with the idea, then at least do one breastfeed, she'll benefit hugely even from that.

So now that you're going to breastfeed, this is what you do. Take my number, ring anytime. Feed the baby whenever it needs, and this will get your supply established. When getting help in the hospital, conversationally ask the midwife helping you did she breastfeed her own children and for how long.

If she has never breastfed, be careful of her advice. Try and find a group of like minded mothers, for chat and support. When you have visitors, and they ask "What can I do?" you say, "Will you empty the dishwasher, hang the clothes, buy some food, wash the floor..."

When they ask, "Can I bring something?" You say, "Yes, thanks. If you're passing Superquinn, I need..." and give them a list. This is called getting support.

Get a good book on breastfeeding. Bring it to the hospital. And ring me whenever.

Most of all: Go with your instincts.

Mairead

Chapter Eight

BREASTFEEDING IN IRELAND: PART TWO

I think most pregnant women know that "breast is best." I don't believe that any more education in that regard will help. I think it is still considered a bit odd and that a lot of women are squeamish about it. For the 50% who never even give it a try, I think the only way they will is by seeing more people breastfeeding out and about and by having friends who breastfeed. In other words, seeing it as normal. Hopefully, this will come with time. For the majority of the other 50%, who try it but don't last long, it's all about support. In the hospitals, from the PHN's, from family and friends. They don't even have to be breastfeeding experts, sometimes all you need to hear is "You are doing a great job!" to keep you going.

Shirley, 36, Dublin

Breastfeeding By Numbers in Ireland

Breastfeeding is an unequaled way of providing ideal food for the healthy growth and development of infants; it is also an integral part of the reproductive process with important implications for the health of mothers. As a global public health recommendation, infants should be exclusively breastfed (1) for the first six months of life to achieve optimal growth, development and health. (2) Thereafter, to meet their evolving nutritional requirements, infants should receive adequate and safe complementary foods while breastfeeding continues for up to two years of age or beyond. Exclusive breastfeeding from birth is possible except for a few medical conditions, and unrestricted exclusive breastfeeding results in ample milk production.

World Health Organization (WHO) as stated in the Global Strategy on Infant and Young Child Feeding (WHA55 A55/15, paragraph 10)

Ireland has the lowest rates of breastfeeding in Europe.
55 % of mothers in Ireland initiate breastfeeding at birth.
35% Stop within the first two weeks.
72% of Irish babies are fully formula fed by four months of age.
2.4% of mothers in Ireland are exclusively breastfeeding their babies at 6 months of age as per the recommendations of the WHO (World Health Organization)

81% of mothers in Ireland who had stopped breastfeeding between 3 and 4 months of age would like to have breastfed for longer.

(All Statistics taken from The National Infant Feeding Survey 2008, University of Dublin, Trinity College Dublin School of Nursing and Midwifery - prepared for the HSE by Professor Cecily Begley, Chair of Nursing and Midwifery, Louise Gallagher, Doctoral Student/Midwifery Research Assistant, Dr. Mike Clarke Adjunct Professor TCD and Director of UK Cochrane Center, Margaret Carroll, Director of Midwifery and Sally Millar, Lecturer in Midwifery)

The Pub with no Beer
(Kindly reprinted with author's permission. First appeared in the popular blog, Irish Mammy on the Run.)

As I find five minutes to write, here is the latest update:

Baby Seán is doing well. He's eleven days old now and he has re-gained his ten percent weight loss. He is a total guzzler and sometimes feeds every two hours ... so I'm getting lots of sleep – not.

I have tried everything in the rule book to get breastfeeding, and alas, I have come to accept that it is not meant to be. I have spoken to Cuidiú, I have met with two lactation consultants and I spoke on the phone to a third lady. I bought an electric pub. I was then advised to hire a *hospital* style pump from Cuidiú after which I sent my husband to another county to find the right size 'phlanges'.

I have been drinking fennel tea, pumping religiously every three to four hours. I have been massaging, taking hot showers, doing skin to skin with the baby. I have even tried taking immodium as it is said to stimulate the pituitary gland. Tortured by thoughts that sometimes in c-section patients the milk comes in a little later - normally between days 7 and 10 – I spent days five to ten pumping to no avail.

I was surprised to learn that I actually am a 'bizarre case'. In fact, so strange am I, that my situation was discussed at a lactation consultants association of Ireland meeting this week. They all thought it was 'extremely unusual' that I was determined, pumping, doing skin to skin with the baby and all those other things I mentioned, and still nothing. Basically a few drops (literally drops) over the seven day period but they said I should have been getting something more substantial.

So today I hang up my pumps and admit that I am the pub with no beer. At least I retire from breastfeeding knowing I have done my best. The lactation consultant (who is believed to be number one in Ireland) said I have done everything right. It seems I just fall into the 2% category of 'unexplained cases where the mother does not produce milk.'

Now the search is on to find the underlying problem. Possible scenarios include; cysts, hormonal imbalance or products/placenta part remaining in the uterus.

I have met my fair share of militant midwives, especially in Denmark. I have met a few in Dublin but my preferred midwives are the Irish mothers and the Polish mothers, both of whom were supportive but not shoving it down my throat. In the end, everyone could see I was trying my best. I was even told that I was one of the most perseverant breastfeeding mothers they had ever met. Especially post c-section when every turn/lift and in/out of bed movement hurts. I can only say to those women who insist that every woman can breastfeed, I don't believe it is true.

Now, instead of beating myself up over the VBAC and inability to breastfeed, I am going to focus on what is important, enjoying the first precious moments with my baby.

Real Mams Talk about:
Breastfeeding -Why not?
I was a breast woman until it all went wrong. Now that James is on the bottle and thriving, my negativity towards the bottle is gone. So the choice was made for me. He got the good stuff in the beginning and next time I will try again and won't listen to any doctors about starving babies :(

Fiona, 29, Dublin

I found it very difficult, I was delirious when she would finally latch on, but there were problems. She vomited a lot, and was having trouble feeding. At the midwife's decision she was bottle fed by day three.

Sarah, 28, Cork

I really only made up my mind when I went in to hospital. I really wanted to try breastfeeding but I got a lot of very negative feedback from my family and friends. Actually, not one person encouraged me to breast feed apart from my ante natal classes. I feel like I was misinformed about it. It's one of my big regrets. However, my son as it turns out, is lactose intolerant so it was probably for the best that he was bottle fed on special lactose free formula. Hopefully when I have another baby I will breastfeed.

Emma, 29, Cork

Oh, I'm a bottle woman. I just didn't feel comfortable with the idea of breast feeding, I don't know why. Also, I have to say that I felt I had done my bit for the nine months and bottle feeding meant that my husband could be partly responsible for feeding. my two have thrived on the bottle, they were both great feeders, thank God.

A, 33, Dublin

I breastfed for three days and that was it. The pain was something I wasn't prepared for and after three sleepless nights in hospital I was unable to deal with the pain in my nipples and the pain from labour. Thankfully, she took the bottle no bother but I feel dreadful that I didn't breastfeed for longer. I would hope to breastfeed my next child but would feel guilty if I do it for longer than on the first!

Jennifer, 28, Meath

I started off breastfeeding and it went well. It wasn't sore and she had no problems latching on. As time went on though, I began to resent her constantly wanting feeding. I dreaded feeding time. I hated getting my boobs out! So we gradually switched to formula and the first bottle of it she had, she slept the whole afternoon and then six hours that first night. We were on to a winner! I preferred being able to see how much she was drinking so I had an idea of whether she would be full or not. I have huge admiration and respect for mothers who persevered but it just wasn't for me. If I have another child I will breastfeed for the first while again but will have no problems switching if it isn't working.

Chris, 31, Cork

I tried breastfeeding but sadly, I only lasted two days. Grace was very, very hungry and as I was a first time mother I was getting very anxious so I asked for formula. The midwife looked at me as if I was asking for her blood! Of course I am well informed of the benefits of breastfeeding and I regret not persisting but it just broke my heart to see and hear my little angel crying...

Amanda, 32, Limerick

I chose to bottle feed. I did consider breast feeding but I felt that the bottle was right for me. At least my partner could do night feeds, so no excuses there! I've had no problems and it's good to know exactly how much he's drinking.

Kim, 22, Dublin

I fully intended to breastfeed Philip but he was too lazy. He would not open his mouth enough for the boob! The hospital staff were not a great support. If they had been I might have persevered, but it being all so new and scary, I expressed for two days and then went on to the bottle. When Katie was born I was unsure of breast feeding. I gave it a try in the hospital and she was on for it but I had trouble getting her to latch on, I was told I have flat nipples. Again, the support was not great and I decided it was going to be too difficult trying to breastfeed a baby and look after a demanding toddler so I gave in. : (

Louise, 28, Cavan

With my second child, I had to give up breastfeeding at five weeks as I was hospitalized twice with bad kidney infections and the medication would have been too strong for her. I was very disappointed because I had hoped to do it for another while. It then took another four months to get the right formula, which was quite traumatic for her and extremely exhausting for me.

Elaine, 29, Cork

I started with breastfeeding but as I had a section I found it really hard as your milk takes longer to come in. I decided that bottles were the best decision for me. I do think that on my next child I will try to breastfeed again though. The connection you feel is just amazing. That was the hardest thing for me to let go of when I decided to stop. I felt like I was letting him down. I do think there are upsides to bottle feeding though. I was able to go on a night out after four weeks and had a brilliant time. I also think that it makes your baby more independent and that can be a good thing.

Maria, 25, Dublin

I tried breast feeding but none of the kids latched on. But the good thing about the bottle is that other people can help. My partner enjoyed feeding the babies because he felt it helped him bond.

Mother of Three, Monaghan

Well, this is the one part I do "regret." I feel now that I never pushed myself far enough. I always wanted to breastfeed and after an awful labour (induction, no pain relief for hours etc...) and little to no support from the hospital staff (too busy, not enough staff.) Orlaith ended up latching on wrongly at some stage.

After we got home, it got worse and worse. In the end I was in agony and bleeding. I went to the public health nurse and she told me there was a breastfeeding support group the next day at another health centre. So I went there thinking that the public health nurse would watch how she was latching on and tell me what was going wrong but no....a few other mums were there for their babies to be weighed and basically, she didn't even want me to show her what I was doing. She just told me there was nothing I could do and basically I had to just work through the pain, that it would get better. That night I stopped, after my hubby told me enough was enough when I was sitting there, crying with the pain as she was feeding.

Ruth, 37, Dublin

I call the first two weeks "the dark days." I had a crap time try- ing to breastfeed and felt like I was feeding Harry poison when I gave him his first bottle of formula. In fact, I couldn't do it. My husband had to do it. He'd never latched on and I'd expressed all his feeds for two weeks. My boobs aren't the largest and I only went up to a B cup when I had him so I could just about squeeze out sixty mls in thirty minutes. Everyone kept saying keep going, keep going, it'll get easier. It was my doctor who finally said to give it up. Not demanding, or bossy like. She just saw a new mother with sties on both eyes, ulcers covering her mouth, dark circles and pale skin and realized I was miserable, so was my husband and it had to have been affecting Harry. It was like music to my ears really. I just wanted someone to say it's okay to give up, and she did.

Kirsty, 29, Dublin

Dairine's Story

According to infallible sources such as Grazia magazine, the average woman of my vintage (32) with no health issues should expect to conceive within six months of stepping off the contraception wagon. I added on 2 months for the smoking and then deducted 2 months for being slightly overweight - apparently, in fertility circles this is good – although I suspect that they mean by ounces rather than pounds.

Using this highly scientific reasoning, I deducted that if I stopped taking my pill at the end of December I could still enjoy my Australian holiday in January, knock the last bit of craic out of the drinking and smoking and maybe become pregnant sometime in the summer. With any luck I would be one of those oblivious women who never realized they were pregnant until they were about three months gone, thus avoiding the constant worry of the first twelve weeks.

Of course, Mother Nature had other plans and six seconds later I was knocked up. And no, we weren't at it like rabbits. As I mentioned before, the tummy tickling only happens at the weekends as we are living the Commuter Dream and usually go to bed the minute we get home. In the summer we sometimes fall asleep to the sound of the neighbor's kids playing on the road.

We're not great at magical moments in my house and sharing of the news of our impending arrival was no exception. Not for me the strategic placing of a minuscule babygro with "Daddy's little helper" at his place on the table, no tiny Tipperary jersey offered with a coy smile to the future father. Instead, it was as we are, very matter of fact.

The oblivious Dad to be was out foraging for breakfast while I lazed around our Sydney holiday apartment in a fog of confusion trying to work out the implications of getting the time difference wrong between kilcock (that well known line of longitude) and Sydney and slowly realizing that I was in fact "late." By some time.

Upon his return, laden down with lattes and raisin toast, he barely had time to share the spoils before being requested to, "look at this stick and tell me what you can see"

"Two lines," he said.

"Right," I replied, holding out the instruction manual for his perusal. "Now, tell me which of these two pictures the stick looks like; this diagram of one line or this diagram of two lines"

"Definitely the one of the two lines." His eyes widened as the penny finally dropped. "Sweet divine Jesus we're having a baby."

Of course I was too posh to push as there are few things in life as close to a night in Nobu as a Sunday afternoon C section in Mullingar regional – everyone knows that. The sheer glamour of being dead from the waist down while your husband watches the surgeon remove and replace your internal organs is truly a high point in any lady's life.

Of course no high class occasion would be complete without the requisite haute couture and the ankle to thigh stretchy white support stockings supplied by the HSE truly lived up to my high fashion standards. How unfortunate for my poor husband that the first - and only - time I ever wore suspender stockings, they were white, made from industrial strength stretch elastic and accessorized with any amount of sweat and shuffle fluff from the otherwise immaculate hospital floor.

Of course I had always planned to breastfeed. Breast is best, lose your baby weight, no bottle sterilizing, madonna and child - sign me up. I was well prepared too as I had forked out for private anti natal classes and paid close attention when the woman held a doll up to her bosom and with a deft flick of the wrist created a perfect simulation of the "latching on" magic.

This elusive latching on quickly became the centre of my entire world and that of everyone around me when I completely and utterly failed at it.

The ease with which Dolly had happily latched on to Ms. Ante Natal was sorely misleading, as myself and my new son were soon to discover. The boy nestled, nudged, nosed and eventually fell asleep every single time I attempted to feed him while I became more and more frustrated, tense and hormonal.

Appreciation of all the wonderful things we had already achieved together quickly dissipated. The 8.5 months of stress free pregnancy, the speedy and safe delivery and the miracle of having a healthy baby seemed like nothing if I could not achieve this most "natural"of states. It was, without exception, the hardest thing I had ever tried, and failed, to do.

I appreciate that my perception at the time may have been slightly askew but in the small scale world of those first few days it took on gigantic proportions. Helpful comments about the cows in the field and all those women in Africa did not prove particularly motivating, nor did the helpful input of experienced feeders telling me to just stick at it and it would happen – it didn't.

On and on it went – every two hours we would try to get the boy to stay awake so I could get some food into his tiny tummy and every time he started, stopped, and fell fast asleep. We took off his nappy, tickled his feet, wet his bum with cold water on cotton wool - which I'll never forgive myself for, but we were desperate – all to no avail. And so to the expressing.

One helpful HSE leaflet with a line diagram later and we were off, but even that was far from easy. For the first three days I massaged, kneaded and pummeled my breasts like bread dough, all for a few measly drops of colostrum. The nurses, and even a lactation specialist, couldn't have been more supportive but after days of eking out minuscule drops that wouldn't feed a kitten I eventually hit the pump.

Thankfully at this point any fragile desire to retain any dignity had passed and I was prepared, I thought, to do anything to get things on track while topping up the boy with capfuls of formula. Some people say that this was the undoing of it all, but for us, starving our baby was never an option. I was given a schedule, and what a schedule it was...

Synchronize your watches to noon Greenwich Mean Time and thunderbirds are go!

Attempt feeding for a minimum of 25 minutes to "encourage" baby to feed from the breast.

12.25: Proceed to expressing room with hungry baby and place plastic funnels over breasts. Press start. Listen to Westmeath FM slightly off frequency for 15 minutes. Press stop. Pretend to be elated at the 10mls of milk you have managed to collect in the beaker.

Sterilize equipment and return to room for 1pm. Feed baby with 10mls breast milk topped up with formula which flows effortlessly, like a mountain stream, from the carton, reminding me that I do not.

Do not, under any circumstances, get any sleep, eat properly or stop fretting about the schedule despite constant reminders from "Team Liam" that these are the very things that will help the milk to flow. They're not on the schedule though, so scratch that.

After five days of listening to "Hey Delilah" in Mullingar's milking parlor my struggle with the schedule finally came to an end with a visit from one of the nurses who had been on nights during my sojourn and who popped in to say goodbye.

Anyone who has ever been in hospital always talks about "this one nurse" who really made the difference between what was and what could have been. My Angel of Mercy sat on my bed and asked me how I was feeling . This was of course the one question that whipped away any vestige of restraint I may have had left.. When you feel like the world is against you there is always the will to fight back, but people being nice to you? That's a different matter altogether. Predictably, I wept buckets.

She told me she had watched me go up and down the corridor to the expressing room every two hours for the past week, looking like a zombie and being held up by my rolling cot containing the sleeping boy who wouldn't feed. Then she said the words that cannot be spoken out loud by any self respecting modern, well educated woman,

" You know you don't have to breastfeed. "

I climbed warily back on to my soap box to reiterate why this was not the case but she kept on talking,

" Of course it would be wonderful if it's working out for you. If it's what you really want then keep going but try to keep things in perspective. You're going home today and taking your beautiful, healthy boy home with you. When you get there you'll mind him and love him and never let anything harm him.

'He'll be fine – you'll be fine – you and his Dad will love him with all your hearts –that's what's important, nothing else."

I know she probably shouldn't have said it and I know that if I had tried a little bit harder or for a little bit longer it might all have worked out. But at that time, in that place, I think she might just have said just the right thing.

So we took the boy home - driving at thirty miles an hour with regular stops to check he was still breathing - and out of the structured ways and grueling schedule of the hospital, something happened. I took back control of feeding my baby.

We started getting to know each other better and of course, the nurse was right. We mind him and love him and kiss his toes and tickle his tummy and amazingly we offer him bottles of formula milk and he drinks them!

I don't know if he gets more colds or upset tummies then if I had breast fed him and I don't know if it will be the defining factor in his getting pipped at the post for winning the Nobel prize for nuclear physics. I don't particularly care.

There's really no competition as far as we're concerned – boob fed or bottle fed the result is just the same - our perfect boy wins best in show, every time, all categories.

Breastfeeding twins
– What Happens when One Twin Can't?
When I found out I was expecting twins, I initially thought that my plans to breastfeed would go out the window. But when I talked to other twin mums and read up on it I found that lots of mothers do manage to successfully breastfeed twins and even triplets. I read everything I could on breastfeeding twins, and decided I would aim to breastfeed or mix feed for the first three months.

As my pregnancy progressed, I felt confident that I would be able to give it my best shot at least. What I hadn't considered was that one twin would take to breastfeeding straight away but the other wouldn't. But this is exactly what happened.

As the girls had suffered from severe twin-to-twin transfusion syndrome in the womb, there was a big size difference between them when they were born at 35+6 – Rachel was 6 lbs 4oz, and Sarah was 3 lbs 14 oz. This meant that Rachel spent only one night in NICU whereas Sarah spent 15 nights there. Although

Rachel was very small and sleepy as is common with preemies, she took to breastfeeding very well after the first day and a half and soon learned to latch on well. However Sarah wasn't able to feed at all and had to have tube feeds for the first two weeks.

It really didn't help that the hospital weren't as supportive of breastfeeding as they should have been. I was constantly being pressured to give Rachel formula when she was too sleepy to breastfeed, even though I knew that if I left her a bit longer she would have breastfed happily. And there were no facilities to express – I didn't even have a power point in my cubicle to plug in the breast pump – so I wasn't able to express milk for Sarah until after I got home from hospital.

In NICU the nurses really discouraged me from trying to breast-feed Sarah, saying she was too small. I wanted to do skin-to-skin contact with her to at least get her used to that, but we were told not to take her out of her blankets as she would get cold. I found myself almost surreptitiously putting her to the breast when the nurses weren't looking.

The first couple of weeks were a blur of breastfeeding Rachel, giving her formula top-ups, expressing for Sarah, keeping track of exactly how many mls she was having and storing the milk accordingly (it went from 25 mls to 60 mls in gradual increments of 2-3 mls!), and trying to get in to the hospital to see Sarah at feed time without missing one of Rachel's feeds. We had my mother staying for part of the time but when she went home we had to go to visit Sarah separately, and I couldn't drive after my C-section so I was relying on friends for lifts.

Sarah came off the tube feeds after 13 days and was having formula and EBM (expressed breast milk) from a bottle. We were shocked when we went in to see her on the 16th day and were told we could take her home. Although it was fantastic news, we weren't prepared – we hadn't thought about what bottles we would use for her at home (she couldn't drink from the avent bottles Rachel had – her mouth was too small to get around the teat) and we didn't even have the car seat with us. But it was such an amazing feeling to take her home and be together properly as a family of four for the first time.

I continued trying to breastfeed Sarah as often as I could but she was not a good feeder. Sometimes she would latch on well but come off again after a minute or too. Other times I would spend 15 minutes trying to get her to latch on, or else she wouldn't latch on at all. Even when it seemed like she had fed well, she obviously wasn't taking in as much as her sister, because she would be hungry again within half an hour. I could spend an hour trying to feed her, and then end up giving her a bottle as well or instead. Then it would be time to feed Rachel, and I would have missed out on my chance to express for Sarah until after the next feed. I found myself with the dilemma of wondering whether it was best to keep trying to breastfeed her, or to simply forget it and use the time to express instead, so that at least I could be sure she was getting breast milk.

It used to make me laugh reading advice about breastfeeding twins which went along the lines of 'At the first feed, feed twin one on the left and twin two on the right, then switch over at the next feed'. This assumed that both twins fed at the same time all day long and had the same number of feeds per day. This simply wasn't true for my twins, and if I had attempted to impose a routine on them, I would have been going against the advice to let breastfed babies feed on demand. Everything I read seemed to contradict something else and it was impossible to know what to do for the best.

I sought help everywhere I could think of. I posted on discussion forums specializing in breastfeeding and others specializing in twins. I read five or six different books. I went to the breastfeeding clinic in the hospital where the twins were born. I had a private lactational consultant visit me at home to give me advice. I went to a breastfeeding support group in my local health centre. I tried dozens of different suggestions to try to get Sarah to feed directly from me. Eventually she did manage to breastfeed a bit, but she never became a very good feeder and always needed a top up from a bottle.

After about eight weeks we fell into a routine of sorts. I would breastfeed Rachel all day and she would have formula at bed-time. I would try to breastfeed Sarah once at some point during the day, usually in the morning, but if it didn't work we just moved on. I expressed for her first thing in the morning, again later in the day, and last thing at night after we put the girls to bed. This worked very well, but I continued to feel sad about the fact that I was 'properly' breastfeeding one twin and not the other. The best piece of advice I got at this time was from a friend who said to me 'but you're feeding each baby in the way that's right for her'.

It was true. Although breast milk is of course the best thing you can give your baby, continuing to try to breastfeed Sarah was clearly not in her best interests as she got so tired and frustrated, and at least by expressing for her she was getting the breast milk anyway.

At first I felt like I was the only person who had ever been in this position. It was impossible to give a simple answer when people asked 'Are you breastfeeding them?'. But when I talked to other twin mums I did find some who had been in a similar position. One had decided to stop breastfeeding altogether. One had decided to stop breastfeeding directly but had continued to express for both twins for a few months. She said she felt it was fairer as she didn't like the fact that she was spending more time with the breastfed twin, but in retrospect she was sorry she hadn't continued to breastfeed as it would have kept her supply going for longer. One had done similar to myself and mainly breastfed one, with the other having occasional breast-feeds when he could manage it. One had been unable to express but had continued to breastfeed the 'good' feeder and the other had been fully formula fed.

In the midst of the guilt of being unable to 'properly' breastfeed Sarah, I found myself wondering how things would have been different if she hadn't been a twin. Maybe if I had been able to be there for all her feeds when she was in NICU and tried to breastfeed her every time she needed a feed, instead of just when I wasn't feeding Rachel, then she might have learnt to breastfeed better. On the other hand, if she hadn't had a twin sister keeping my supply going I might have stopped expressing for her much sooner and she wouldn't have had the benefit of so many months of breast milk. It's impossible to know, but as mothers we do like to beat ourselves up over these things!

I continued to breastfeed/ mix feed until the girls were 5 months old. By then I had really come to hate expressing and found it getting increasingly painful. Although I was still enjoying breastfeeding, I decided it was time to stop as I couldn't give one baby breast milk and not the other.

Looking back on my breastfeeding experience, I'm so glad I managed to breastfeed Rachel and express for Sarah for as long as I did. Although I'll always be a bit sad that I couldn't fully breastfeed both, I have no regrets and know that I did the best I could – which is all any of us can do!

Real Mams Talk About:
Breastfeeding in Ireland – Why the Low Rates?

I think most pregnant women know that "breast is best." I don't believe that any more education in that regard will help. I think it is still considered a bit odd and that a lot of women are squeamish about it. For the 50% who never even give it a try, I think the only way they will is by seeing more people breast-feeding out and about and by having friends who breastfeed. In other words, seeing it as normal. Hopefully, this will come with time. For the majority of the other 50%, who try it but don't last long, it's all about support. In the hospitals, from the PHN's, from family and friends. They don't even have to be breastfeeding experts, sometimes all you need to hear is "You are doing a great job!" to keep you going.

Shirley, 36, Dublin

Breastfeeding is not in our culture here. As stated at the top of this questionnaire, even baby dolls come equipped with bottles. For some reason it is far more acceptable to bottle feed than breastfeed. Hunger in a baby is synonymous with wanting a bottle. It is probably a result of a combination of extremely suc-cessful marketing by the formula companies and the ingrained perception of breasts only as sexual objects. Probably as a re-sult of this last - because I am not a prude! Really!! - I have bat-tled with this notion myself the past eight months. I still can't tell people I "breastfeed." Instead, I tell them I am, "feeding her myself" so that I don't have to say the word "breast" out loud. (Truly)

I think the health service here is no great shakes at getting rates up either, but I see that no matter how supportive they were, they would have a job to change an entire culture! It is the likes of gradually more and more of us girls quietly and publicly doing our thing, having the confidence to feed our babies the way we want to in the face of a deeply established culture of bottle feeding that will eventually turn the tide. And the more of us who do it, the bigger the base of support that experienced breast feeders can provide to new mammies. As the first of my peers to have a baby, I came to it having nobody close to me that I could ask for help or advice in the early days. I am happy now that I will be there to provide the personal support I was deprived of when they go on to have babies.

Adrienne

There are so many reasons. Culturally, we have so quickly normalized bottle feeding. Our mums were coerced - along with almost their entire generation - into formula feeding and their generation is one of the loudest voices saying, "but you were formula fed and you turned out fine." We need as a culture to get over ourselves. We need to say, "yes, we were misled, and now it's time to fix it."

Advertising of formula with all its shiny happy families needs to be stopped. It perpetuates the myth that formula is as good as breastfeeding, and it's not. It might be an essential choice for some mothers or a lifestyle choice for others, but it should be an informed choice, not one that is made because of some glossy ads.

But more than that, our government needs to step up to the mark. In Ireland, most mums have to work outside the home to pay hefty mortgages and fathers don't even get one day - let alone a few weeks – paternity leave after the baby is born! This puts a lot of pressure on mothers to go against the flow, often on their own. The HSE is woefully inadequate, PHN (public health nurse) advice is all over the place and the vast amount of GPs still advise solids at four months and ask, "are you still breastfeeding?" with a look of shock on their faces!

At the end of the day though, it is everyone's personal responsibility to educate themselves and their children in the normal functioning of the human body. Breasts are not just for selling cars!

Kate, 31, Galway

A lot of Irish people seem to think that there is something disgusting about breastfeeding and that attitude needs to be addressed. I think more independent breastfeeding help needs to be out there. The HSE pay lip service to "Breast is Best" but when it comes down to it, no one is quicker to give the baby a bottle then some of the midwives and doctors. I also think that young mums need lots of support. I'm a young mum and my friends think it's gross and why would I want to burden myself? Even the doctors and midwives thought because of me being a young mum I would find it too hard.

Lucretia, 20, Dublin

Culture. And love of bloody bottles. I think that there's a culture here of, "What's all the fuss about children? Just feed them and get on with everything." There is a lack of recognition that love, cuddles, touch and time are as important as food and shelter.

Also, it comes form the top, medical staff don't seem to realize the importance of breastfeeding. And this pride about children being independent! I don't understand why people think this early independence is a good thing. They are children. They're not supposed to be independent and we're not supposed to be able to "get on with everything." We should cherish being able to teach and nurture them, and of course, feed them properly.

To improve rates seems to be very difficult. We do need more support, a lot more, but I think there has to be a fundamental mind-shift in the importance of infant nutrition. Something like, "If you have a baby you breastfeed unless you really can't."

I don't believe breastfeeding needs to be medicalized but because most babies are born in hospitals I think medical staff have to be - I hate to use the word but feel I have to - aggressively educated. And I speak as a health professional who is appalled at my own lack of education on the matter. And I was always pro breastfeeding, so you can imagine the education for health professionals not interested in breastfeeding. This is a massively important issue. Then let it filter down.

And keep it public. Public, public, public! Emphasize the importance of breastfeeding. None of this "advantages of bottle feeding" stuff. It really irritates me. There are no advantages. Stronger control on infant formula advertising, also really irritates me. No more automatic infant formula in hospitals. You know, no trolley with a nurse going, "breast or bottle?" In times to come, I bet we'll be appalled at that. Kind of like the cigarette ladies of old with their, "would you like a cigarette?"

Mairead

More promotion by the HSE, obviously to pregnant women, but also in the national media so that the wider population, which includes grandparents to be and other relatives and friends who may not have breastfed, to understand the benefits. Inclusion in the secondary school curriculum, perhaps in home economics, so that the correct information is disseminated at an early age rather than some of the misconceptions people may have. More breastfeeding mums feeding in public so that it is not seen as anything to be hidden away.

Muriel, 33, Dublin

Friends of Breastfeeding
Friends of Breastfeeding are a voluntary organization that was formed by a group of mothers who met on online parenting forums. Many of these mothers found the Internet to be the only place they could access true support and reliable information and advice about breastfeeding. The need for two things was clear to everyone involved - better understanding of breastfeeding across the general public, and improved access to good breastfeeding support in Ireland for women who want to breastfeed their babies. Friends of Breastfeeding work to ensure that women in Ireland achieve their desired breastfeeding experience. We network to connect women in Ireland who want to breastfeed with their local support system. We work to build

communities of supportive friends, family and health professionals - "friends" of breastfeeding.

The whole concept of 'Friends' of Breastfeeding is that we are not exclusively a group of breastfeeding mothers. We welcome anyone who recognizes the importance of breastfeeding. You don't have to breastfeed or even know anyone who does to be a 'Friend'. Research shows that Dads and maternal grandmothers in particular play a major role in a mother having the breastfeeding experience she wants. How you would like to be involved is entirely up to you, we invite people to put themselves forward for anything that might help breastfeeding mothers to have the breastfeeding experience they would choose to have.

Friends of breastfeeding is a registered charity - CHY19054

For more information go to_www.friendsofbreastfeeding.ie_
Email: friendsofbreastfeeding@yahoo.ie

Chapter Nine

POST NATAL DEPRESSION

There is definitely not enough information about PND available to mothers and it is a lot more common than we are led to believe. We are told by all the books and by other women that it is the greatest experience of your life to give birth and that you should immediately feel a bond and this incredible love for your child, that you will be a perfect mother and know it all straight away. This may be the case for many women but not for all and there is a lot of guilt and shame if you don't feel this straight away.

Jennifer, 36

A little Rant...

When I first found out I was pregnant, I had this image in my head - probably from somewhere circa 1956 - of all these new mothers doing motherly things together, like having a chat while hanging the laundry or stopping by for tea while the babies are playing or even just walking together. I imagined this giant, fantastic motherland, and instead discovered that it's more like each of us are quinny buzzing about on our own little islands with our own little babies, totally independent of each other.

We expect ourselves to get back in shape, keep the house immaculate, be perfect mothers to our babies and perfect wives to our husbands/partners and for some women the challenge also extends to being perfect back in the workplace as well. All of this and we are still not getting a good night's sleep and our hormones are all over the place.

When my daughter was about six months old, we were on one of our regular trips to the in-laws. Being the nice person/fool that

I am, I had spent the morning keeping the world spinning on it's axis while I let my darling partner have a lie in (?!?!?!??!?!?!)

That afternoon, I asked him to do a quick job for me on the computer. Halfway through, he disappeared. When I went looking for him, he was upstairs playing on the XBOX with his brother. Being the mature, reasonable person that I am, I threw the laptop down on the bed next to him and in that horrible, icy, very controlled "I am so mad I could kill you" kind of way, said,

"FINE! DO IT WHENEVER IT SUITS YOU THEN!!!!!"

Which all led of course, to him looking at me in that really concerned, "Oh my god....who are you and what have you done with my partner?" sort of way and asking, "Are you alright baby?" Which drives me nuts because... (Drum roll please!)

I am not all right. I am tired. My hair is falling out in clumps and I haven't slept through the night in over a year. There is a very small person who in a very short period of time has eclipsed everyone and everything else in my life to become the most important and loved being in my world. She relies on me for everything and I want to do my best for her. Did I mention that I grew her inside of my uterus, carried her for nine months and then pushed her out through my vagina after an eleven hour labour hooked up to a pitocin drip with antibiotics that made me spend the first few minutes of her life throwing up in a cardboard basin?

I also want to live in a clean house. Not insanely clean, just tidy enough so that it feels as though things are in order. I have lost forty pounds in seven months which is a lot by any standards. I'd love to have the energy to feel sexual but most nights I'd give anything to simply get a full night's sleep. Add to that the fact that the small one seems to spend half the day attached to my breast and is it any wonder I just want five minutes to call my body my own? I would love to "just cuddle" but the only men god invented who can do that are gay!

In the span of fifteen months, my entire world has been turned upside down and inside out. My body was surrendered to nature and I have had to re evaluate every aspect of who and what I am and what is important to me. On top of all that, there is now this tiny piece of skin below my belly button that looks as though it belongs to a ninety year old woman that I have been told every woman who has ever been pregnant possesses and you know what?

I don't mind. I really don't mind all of that.

What I do mind is when my partner leaves towels on the floor after a shower instead of hanging them up to dry, or when I have to ask him for help to do dishes or other chores around the house. I want him to do these things because to me, when he doesn't, it's like a slap in the face. It's as though all the work I put into keeping everything going, means nothing. I guess I just don't understand how he can so easily relax and kick back with the computer or a book or the TV when there is laundry to be washed, dishes to be done and rooms to be tidied.

You are not alone in feeling like the world has tilted off it's axis. I love my life. I honestly do. But I still have days when I scream into my pillow out of sheer frustration or when I start crying and laughing (simultaneously) at the slightest provocation. And you know what? I just know that someday, it's all going to get better. One day, my hair will stop falling out, I will shed those last few pounds, I will regularly sleep through the night and I will look at household chores as just that, household chores, and not as a symbol of my self- worth.

And on that day, I will find out I am pregnant...

Post Natal Depression
It is estimated that around 60 - 70% of women will experience feelings of significant struggle at some point in the first six months after giving birth. To be perfectly honest, I've yet to meet a mother who hasn't. For most new mothers, these feelings are short lived. They reach out to family and friends for support and as the days go by, their confidence grows and life goes on.

Sometimes though, the feelings don't go away. They stay. They linger on and eat away at you. They sap the color and joy out of what you'd thought was going to be the greatest experience of your life. Post Natal depression is thought to effect 20% of women in the first year after giving birth. It's most severe form is known as puerperal psychosis, which effects 1 in 500 new mothers and requires medical care asap.

You are not alone. You did not "fail." PND is nothing to be ashamed of. You can get help and you can get better. The following are stories of Irish mothers who have experienced PND and have been kind enough to share their experiences here.

Sam's Story
In March 2007, we found out we were expecting our first baby. We had only been trying a short time, so we were delighted. The pregnancy was fine except for some pretty bad morning sickness. We spent all that summer preparing and getting very excited about our new arrival. All I wanted was to be a mum and I could not wait to meet our baby.

On November 20th, I had our baby boy Alexander. It was a totally natural birth and I immediately started breastfeeding. I spent two nights in hospital. As I'd had Alexander during the night, by the time I got home I had already had three nights with very little sleep! I did not like being in hospital and got very conflicting information regarding the care and feeding of my baby. This was hard for me as a first time mother, as I did not know who to listen to. Looking back I should have trusted my own instincts, but I was too scared.

Alexander had colic and after a week of breastfeeding, still would not latch on. I expressed for a week but drove myself mad trying to keep up feeding him. After another week, I gave up. I believe that my failure to breastfeed was a huge factor in my PND.

I was very much in love with Alexander, but felt constantly on edge. I could not sleep, I barely ate and after three weeks, I was even lighter that I had been before getting pregnant. It was coming up to Christmas and all my family were coming home for the holidays; so basically, I was firing on all cylinders pretending to love being a mum. I could not tell people I was falling apart. Besides, at that early stage, people would assume that it was just the baby blues.

It was January that I finally cracked. I hated seeing my husband going to work; I wanted to beg him to stay at home with me. I went to the doctor for the baby's and my six week check up - it was a bit late because of Christmas – anyway, I broke down in the doctor's surgery and told him how I felt. He diagnosed me with depression and prescribed medication for me. My husband made arrangements to work from home for a bit and the next day I started my medication.

Unfortunately, I had a bad reaction to the pills and was ill for a few days. My husband went back to work and I decided that I did not need the medication - I could get over this myself. We went to stay with my parents for two weeks and I got some well needed rest. When I felt stronger we went back home.

For another month, I carried on pretending I could do this. Alexander took over every minute of my life. He was a bad sleeper and he had colic, so I never really ventured out at night. I would get out and about during the day to meet other mums but I would always be pretending that everything was okay. I was so sleep deprived that half the time I was going around in a daze. What made things worse for me was that my best friend had her second baby two months before me and she just got in with it.

I was so angry that I was feeling like this and that my life was gone. I would be in my Pajamas by six in the evening and would run around cleaning and tidying. Then I would go to bed and lie awake for hours.

In late February, I had a total meltdown. I phoned my poor mum at work crying and begging for help. She took me back to the doctor and I got different medication this time. We stayed with them for three weeks and things did start to get a bit better. My wonderful husband then planned a lovely holiday for us in April.

Alexander has always been a hard baby in that he does not need much sleep. I love my sleep so again, the sleep deprivation made my depression worse. I stayed on my medication till August 2007, after which I gradually weaned off and then started back to work (I worked from home.)

After two months, I had another minor breakdown and had to stop working. I am currently on sick leave and am still very depressed. I plan to go back on my medication.

I was lucky to have great support from family and friends, I still do. Without them I would have never coped. I do still mourn my old life and I miss the person I was. I know that when you become a mum you have to change but I did not just change, I disappeared. I really want some of the old me back for my husband and my little boy. I am very positive about the coming year. I want to enjoy my little boy now. For the majority of his life so far I have been depressed. I cannot imagine hav-

ing another child as I do not think that I could go through this
again.

I think the main message to any mums who think they have
PND would be to please talk to someone and get treated. Most
people think it will just go away. It doesn't. You need to do
something about it. Every day I ask why did I get this? Why
can't I just be a happy, loving mum? I know I always put my
little boy first and I give him all he needs but I wish he knew the
old, confident happy Sam.

Christiane's Story

My son Liam Joseph was born on July 18th 2005. I had an
emergency section and he was born a healthy 9.5 lbs.

Looking back I realize now that things weren't right from the
start but I put it all down to being tired and exhausted after my
operation. Liam was a big, strong baby with a big appetite! I
was breastfeeding him as well so I thought I just felt worn out.

Myself and my partner were quite young, this baby wasn't
planned and we had no family living nearby. My family lives
abroad and my partner's family are a two hour drive away.
None of our friends had children.

The public Health Nurse did come to our house two or three
times after Liam was born and each time we had a list of questions which she did answer but it was obvious she was under
severe pressure and trying to visit as many families as possible.
No one ever asked how we are coping or how I was feeling,
which is scary really, to think that anyone can have children
and get sent home from hospital with one or two visits and that
is it.

So we just got on with things, I had to return to work after
four months and was lucky to get a part time position. But that
meant that I was working evenings and weekends till late and

I was up with Liam again early in the morning. I was basically tired for two years!

When Liam was about nine months old I brought him to my GP because he had a cold. When sitting in the waiting room I was browsing through some leaflets that were on display. One of them asked a few questions at the front of the leaflet – and I answered all of them with yes! When I turned the page it said that if you answer yes to all or most of the questions you could be suffering from Depression. And it hit me then that that is actually what is wrong with me!

So we went in to see the GP, and when she asked how I was, I just broke down crying so hard. I felt like such a failure as a mother!!! I was so upset but at the same time I was relieved to know there is a name to all of this, it is an illness and I can be cured. I told my GP how bad I feel and like I am not doing a good job and she pointed out that I have a gorgeous, healthy boy sitting on my lap- the picture of happiness. Well, I didn't see it like that I just felt so low.

I was put on Anti Depressants (lustral) which started to help me after a few weeks of taking them. My GP also advised me to do Counseling once I was feeling better. The tablets cost around sixty Euro per month and money was tight in our house at the time so this was another pressure put on me. I feel that medication like this should be given free – I was tempted more than once to not get the tablets as I had no money.

I eventually did do the counseling but had to pay fifty euro for each visit. I did eight sessions but again money was the main reason why I stopped going. The counseling did help in the sense that I talked through the horrible, horrible experience in the maternity ward in Galway. It also helped me to understand that I was probably depressed in the past but never realized it.

I think that the awful stay in the hospital and getting no support from the staff in the Maternity ward was definitely a contributing factor in my depression. I was wrecked after the operation but was told to look after my son who was a heavy baby. If I could have just gotten a good night's sleep it would have made everything easier!

Also, I have a complicated relationship with my own mother and I was afraid history would repeat itself with me and my own son. I just wanted to do a better job than my own mother. When I was at my lowest, I felt like a failure and a bad mother. I thought that Liam didn't like me. I was convinced he could see right through me and what an awful person I was.

I didn't get support from friends and family - partly cos they were all far away, but mainly because I didn't tell anyone. I was ashamed. I only told them afterwards. They were shocked and had no idea what I'd been going through. There was no support in my community. Eventually I found the PND.ie board and got some support from there.

I tried to set up a support group for the West of Ireland, but it never took off. I met a couple of times with another mother I had met through PND.ie though and that helped. Talking is so good. Like everything in life, it is great to be able to share your experience with someone who has been there as well.

I gradually got better and after a year and a half, I weaned off my tablets and have never looked back!

Samantha's Story
The early days? Well, I loved it! I was a first time mum and I was so proud of her! But I soon became very protective of her-I wouldn't let anyone hold her/feed her etc... This gradually became severe post natal depression. She got colic and it was hell!!! Non stop screaming from about 4:00pm till midnight and nothing would stop it.

This went on for about 3months and so I sank deeper and deeper into my depression. No one knew, though my husband eventually started to cop on that something wasn't right but I kept it well hidden. I often thought of ending it all and even harming my precious daughter (even though she was my world) God it was awful!

I never once admitted it or asked for help. I just learned to deal with it I think. I suffered right through until finally when I was three months pregnant on my next baby I went and asked for help! It was the hardest thing I've ever had to do. I was straight away put on tabs and things got better. But I'm still in them to this day.

My second baby is now a year old but I've had the year from hell. When she was two weeks old I discovered my hubby had been cheating on me through my whole pregnancy (with an 18yr old might I add-he's 35!!) So to be honest my tabs and my gorgeous girls are whats kept me going and kept me sane-well kind of sane ha ha. I'll come off them eventually....

Emily's Story
I think I knew pretty much straightaway. I convinced myself it was baby blues. At eight weeks post-birth, I gave up breast-feeding as I was so low and I blamed the breastfeeding for it. I wasn't getting any more than three hours sleep in any twenty four hour period and I thought that if someone could bottle-feed, then I would get some rest. At twelve weeks, I went to see the doc. I was at an all time low.

I always thought someone with post natal depression would look like they had lost the will, you know, like laying in bed all day, never getting dressed and having little or no interest in their baby.

I lived on my nerves and was suffering with extreme anxiety all the time, hence the panic attacks. I was up, dressed, make-up on, hair done, house clean and everything sterilized by 10:00 every morning wondering what to do for the rest of the day.

I wasn't eating and I wasn't sleeping. No one was allowed to mind my daughter and no one was allowed to clean her bottles. Only I could do it.

No-one ever offered me any help as I looked like superwoman from the outside. I am very attached to my daughter; people comment on it like it's a bad thing. Nothing would have prepared me for the vulnerability that comes with parenthood. She's like my heart out there being passed around on plate to people with very jittery fingers (or that's how I saw it). It leaves you wide open, I don't think I will ever sleep properly again to be honest.

If my DH was to describe the signs of pnd, as in my case he would say:

Over-sensitivity, crying at the drop of a hat
Paranoia
Erratic moods, short tempered
Insomnia
A constant need for perfection
A complete inability to switch off......ever!!

My feelings on me: I felt like I had no self worth. I've never felt so unattractive. I find that you become faceless behind a buggy. It's like people don't see you anymore. I was paranoid. I talked about suicide to my husband. I said that my daughter would be better off growing up without me and that with me out of the way, my husband and the grandmothers could rear her and everyone would be happy that I was out of the way.

My feelings towards my daughter: I've always tried to be the best I can with my daughter, I believe I've great time for her and great patience with her. We both interact with her as much as we can and I decided to be a stay at home mom, so she would have consistency in her days. The only thing that concerns me is that my depressed nature will affect her. I leave the room when I cry because even at six months old, I could see her expression change when I cried. I've read this book called, "The Mother Factor" and it explained how children feel responsible for their mum being unhappy. Your upset may never be directed toward them but still they take on the burden...... this frightened the life out of me. I don't want her growing up with a depressed mother. I always think that she's got a raw deal and so it's another thing to beat myself up over.

My feelings toward my DH: In the beginning I resented him going to work on a daily basis. It hit home that his life hadn't changed as much as mine. That he had an outlet every day while I was stuck at home with the baby. He'd be talking about work and stuff, and I had nothing interesting to say anymore. The last year has made me realize that I am married to the kindest, most patient man alive. I adore him and do not know why he sticks around. I know I wouldn't want to come home to me every day!!!!! Physically, things are far from okay, but I've been told that this is the norm for awhile with babies in the house.

On Support: I didn't receive any real support from family or friends, but I think that was my own doing. I've never asked for help and have constructed a wall around myself. I'm a very proud person and would find it impossible to admit I was finding things tough. Both sets of parents have their own lives and help on an occasion. I've no adult sisters and my friends live miles away, so I felt pretty much alone. My GP prescribed meds and going to a mother and toddler group - Standard advice. It was my husband who found me a counselor for PND who I am still attending seven months later. I also found rollercoaster (an Irish parenting site) to be amazing. I posted a thread on baby blues and the amount of messages I received was shocking, blowing the one in five statistic out of the water.

On Contributing Factors: Exhaustion was the main one. I had a c section and I had no privacy in the beginning. I never ever got to nap during the day. People always called to visit without a phone call first. I was shattered and very angry with my husband for not protecting me and the baby. My daughter was like "pass the parcel" for the first six weeks. Everyone wants a piece of the baby and nobody cares about the new mum or her well-being. I have seen this in other cases too. People sat on my couch all day holding my baby while I made tea and sandwiches for them. Even my own parents were all about the baby and forgot about their own child's well being. I was so angry at my nearest and dearest that counseling was the only way to go.

By the time my daughter was twelve weeks old, I was on my knees with exhaustion. She's not a sleeper. Even now, at almost eleven months, I can swear that I have never once napped during the day. That whole, "sleep when the baby sleeps" theory, makes my blood boil. Expectant mothers should be made aware that this may not happen.

My in-laws, the men, were not comfortable with me breastfeeding and would stand outside until I had finished. Even in hospital they would stand outside the cubicle. This was so much pressure for me and I feel so angry when I think about it now. Needless to say, when I'm breastfeeding next time they won't be let past the front door.

I never felt looked-after, even after the section. I was working all the time. And if you find no support coming your way then you have to ask for it. I wish I had told people I needed help. I wish I had told them to get off their arses and make me some lunch while I fed my baby.

Dealing with Depression: I first tried anti depressants but they didn't agree with me. I was very upset about being on meds, so I started counseling instead. I read tons of books and found that being part of a support site such as Rollercoaster really helps. I also stay away from sugar and caffeine – they fuel depression.

I'm much improved now but not entirely over my depression. I still attend counseling once a month. We never get out, so I've no social interaction. With my daughter turning one soon, I've decided that I need to go back to work, even for just two days a week. I crave adult company and we're all agreed that my depression won't go until I take back something for myself. Myself and my husband have also decided that we will get out one night a month. I think that through your own self-help and motivation you can beat depression.

Catherine
I am not sure when I realized it was PND but I knew something was wrong within hours of my baby's birth. First off, my husband was holding our little one in the labour ward and I kept asking him who owned him. I had no recollection of having had the baby. I did not want to hold him. I was crying and crying and quite not with it. I went to the post natal ward and held my baby because I was made to, but I didn't want to. I begged the staff to take my newborn from me that night because I wanted to sleep.

When they came back with him the next morning, I didn't even listen when they told me what he had drank. I just sat in my bed and cried. I kept ringing my husband telling him to come and take the baby. He could not come. I changed him just about but if he got sick it was an effort to change him again.

I felt completely withdrawn from him. I lay in bed crying with my headphones on so I did not have to be aware that he was there. My husband came in and went mad that I was ignoring our son. I didn't care. I sat up in bed screaming at him that I needed something to help me relax and that I was not taking care of "that thing."

My husband told the staff that I was unwell. They said they would get a doctor to see me. I did not see the doc until the next day. He gave me some xanex and said he would call the hospital psychiatrist. I got to see the psychiatrist that day, a Friday. He said that I appeared very unwell and he wanted me to stay in hospital over the weekend until he could review me again.

On Saturday evening I started saying that I wanted to leave. The sister in charge said it would be best for me to stay but I said I was going. I did stay, but later when she left, I dressed myself in my day clothes, took all my stuff, put the baby in his cot, walked to the nurse's station and said to the nurse, "I am leaving now, I do not want this baby. Please take him."

I walked on and she screamed at me and I mean screamed! She said to come back and take this baby right now and to mind him and don't even think of saying a thing like that again. I was so confused that I did as I was told.

After everything I have been thru since the birth I have to say this is the worst memory. All staff in my opinion should be aware of what's going on with each woman on the unit and should be aware of how they are feeling. I was not well and I could have done anything to my baby. Thankfully I did no; but the staff were not in any way helpful. I discharged myself on Sunday morning saying I was fine and wanted to go home. I was far from fine.

My feelings towards myself were very bad for a long time to follow. It was almost two years before I felt myself again. I hated my husband and we broke up in the end. My first child, I adored. I loved him and kissed him and did everything with him but I would not go near my second born. I really hated him. It took over two years but I finally accepted that he was my son. He has just turned three now and he is my darling baby. Sometimes I look at him and can't believe I was not there for him as a baby. I was not a mother to him.

I have to say that support was not great. My GP sent me to hospital when my baby was twelve days old and I was put on Suicide watch. I just wanted to end my life. I was eventually referred to local services and the service was awful. It wasn't until two years later that I met a doctor in the public system who gave me her time and recommended a nurse for me to see twice a week.

I have since worked out my feelings. It took two years and a number of suicide attempts for this to happen. I was on a lot of medication. I am still on meds and I don't know if I will ever stop them but I only see a doctor every four or five months now.

Unless you have suffered from Post Natal Depression, you don't know what it is like. People don't want to know. They want you to get on with it, to mind your baby and yourself and not complain. When it goes on as long as it did with me, they give up on you and don't listen anymore.

There definitely needs to be more public awareness of PND and support for people who suffer. The development of a mother and baby unit is needed. There was meant to be a new one opening in St. Vincent's in Dublin but it never went ahead. A service like this may be of help. I know that I could have benefited from this anyhow. GP's need more awareness as do PHNs. There needs to be more training in maternity hospitals and for staff to be aware when there appears to be a problem.

Jennifer's Story
I was feeding my son every three hours and began having trouble sleeping, especially at night between feeds. I felt very anxious about something happening to my baby. At the end of the fifth week, I was exhausted and was still trying to do everything myself. At this point, I began to have intrusive thoughts about myself and my son and began to feel very spaced out and detached from everything that was going on around me.

This terrified me and at the beginning of week six, I went to my doctor who prescribed a low level of anti depressants to begin with.

My Partner was very supportive and came to the doctor with me. On the Tuesday, I had a bad panic attack when my partner was in work and went to my mam's and explained how I was feeling. My partner had to go away on business for two nights then, so I stayed with my mam and felt progressively worse as the week went on. I had myself 100% convinced that I was going to hurt my son and was terrified to be in the same room as him.

On the Friday morning, my sister, who is a nurse, intervened. She rang the Coombe hospital and spoke with their psych team who referred me back to my doctor for an immediate assessment. Myself and my partner then went to the doctor who put me on calmers and suicide watch and rang to have a place for me in St John of gods hospital in Stillorgan, Dublin.

It is really hard to write about that time in my life as I was really in a bad way and it seems unreal that I was so out of it that I couldn't even look at my own baby. I really wasn't even capable of dressing myself or communicating with anyone. I was admitted that Saturday and spent seven weeks there.

Thankfully, with excellent care from my consultant and his team, I was able to make the transition home and begin bonding with my beautiful son. It has been a very hard road since January 2008, but I am doing much better now. I am still on anti d's and see a psychologist once a month. These, combined with regular exercise and not taking on too much in work or at home, and I am definitely getting there, thank god!

Sonia's Story

After my daughter was born, I knew that baby blues could happen and I was expecting it. What I wasn't expecting was the length of time that they would last. After a month, I couldn't take myself out of the feeling I had and my Mum rang my GP and asked her about it. My GP asked me to come in and see her and she diagnosed PND.

As I was breastfeeding at the time, I didn't get medication but a lot of support from my family and my GP. She would ring me once a week to see how I was. My problem wasn't my child, it was everything else. I couldn't do enough for my child and I did bond with her and I loved being a Mum. What I couldn't take was the isolation and home life that came with it.

I am used to commuting four hours daily to work, meaning that fourteen hour days are the norm for me. I love my job and I found it very hard to be away from it. I didn't have many friends with children and my husband worked longer hours than myself, seven days a week. As my GP said at the time, I was more isolated than a single mum. The reason being that I had a husband, so people left me alone to enjoy my new found motherhood; not realizing that he didn't take time away from work or get to come home early. The only time he took off was to collect us from the hospital. My Mum was fantastic but I felt guilty, as she too had her own life and her own job.

In my opinion, I don't think I really ever got over it, it just got easier and I just got used to it. I now have a second new born baby. I worried that I would be in trouble again but so far I'm doing good. I think what contributed to that is that my baby was in special care for a month after being born and is still being checked to see what the problem is so I'm in and out of appointments every week and the first month I practically lived in the hospital as I was breastfeeding also.

I'm not sure how other Mum's coped, I didn't know anyone else with it and I didn't know where to find people with it to talk to. I find now that websites like Rollercoaster are great for meeting people like myself and talking. I just wish I had found it at the time.

Anonymous
Despite longing for a baby, and planning the pregnancy, the shock to the system of of caring for the baby was unreal. I was lucky enough to have a nice easy pregnancy. Although I had previously miscarried and was constantly worrying about the baby, I never had any complications thankfully.

Unfortunately the birth and days following were very traumatic. I had a long labour which resulted in a birth by suction and forceps, leaving both me and the baby physically and mentally wrecked. The hospital staff were overstretched so I had to manage on my own with very little support and no rest/sleep for the first few days, which meant I never got a chance to recover.

It (the depression) probably started as soon as my son was born, but as there was very little mention of PND in any of the antenatal classes I attended or in the books I read, I didn't know what it was or what to do. I was so confused and ashamed of myself that I didn't get help until ten months later.

I firmly believe that the main contributing factor in my depression was the terrible pressure put on me to breastfeed, and unfortunately, my failure to be able to do so. I was put under immense pressure by the staff at the hospital and the public health nurse, and my own mother, and all my friends were breastfeeding at the time. I thought it would be easy, so when it didn't work out I felt like a total failure.

I was so determined I expressed milk for six weeks and then finally, when my body and spirit gave up, I stopped and switched to bottles. It was something I should have done a long time before, but I didn't have the courage to stand up to the nurses and I didn't want to admit defeat I suppose. Even though I eventually gave up and was much happier with a happier baby, I think the damage was done, and my confidence as a mother was smashed because I couldn't do this one simple thing for him.

I felt like a failure, a bad mother, that everyone else was coping better than me, I hope it hasn't affected my son, who's now twenty months, but I'm sure he picked up on my stress and anxiety and panic at trying to carry out the simplest of tasks. My husband and I fought constantly for ten months until I finally caved in and explained how I was feeling. He did his best to support me and was shocked that he had never noticed how bad I had gotten. He found it very hard to deal with me when I was in 'a state' but did his best. Unfortunately there is even less support for partners of PND sufferers.

My GP was fantastic and really helped me out by chatting to me and helping me understand that it was normal and common to feel like this and that she had treated lots of women for the same thing. She also put me on mild medication for a few months. She still always asks how I am. I also went back to work part time, which definitely helped me feel human again.

I didn't tell any of my friends as I was and still am slightly embarrassed, and I suppose I don't want them know that I 'failed' to cope. I told the people that mattered, and that needed to know. My mother was the best support, although I didn't expect her to understand, being from a different generation, but she was so sorry she hadn't been there more for me and told me she though I was managing so well with the baby that she should not interfere, when in fact I needed her to 'interfere' more..... My mother in law on the other hand, just dismissed me, and I regret telling her at all.....

Now, when I feel a bad day coming on, I try and take a deep breath, and tell myself I can cope. If I'm really not coping, I call my mam and she helps me out for the day. I also make sure I have lots of things to do. I organize activities with my son like swimming, Gymboree etc, and meet up with friends and other mothers as much as possible.

The main thing to help me cope was to stop beating myself up for the little things, and feeling guilty for everything I did or didn't do. For example: if my son is sick or in bad form with teething and I can feel my nerves about to snap, then I let him watch telly for thirty minutes to calm him down give me head space. I also took up a hobby to give me some time out in the evening when my husband gets home from work. My husband and I also have a 'date night' every couple of weeks. We get a baby sitter and go for dinner or to the cinema or even just go for a nice drive and get a bag of chips to restore some sense of normality to our relationship.

I am expecting my second baby now and can already feel it creeping back......perhaps it will always be there, or maybe it never really went away. I am going to see my GP next week.

What do you feel is the public perception of post natal depression in Ireland?
There is definitely not enough information about PND available to mothers and it is a lot more common than we are led to believe. We are told by all the books and by other women that it is the greatest experience of your life to give birth and that you should immediately feel a bond and this incredible love for your child, that you will be a perfect mother and know it all straight away. This may be the case for many women but not for all and there is a lot of guilt and shame if you don't feel this straight away. I think that the public perception of PND is improving. I found from being in hospital that it is viewed differently and more sympathetically than other "mental" illnesses. But people still do tend to brush it under the carpet and in my experience,

talking about it as much and as openly as you can helps to normalize it and reduce the fear and shame around it.

Jennifer, 36

I don't think people really understand the range of PND, from the mildest to the most severe, and just brand it all with the same way. I think my generation (35) are far more interested and so far more aware in things like PND. I'm not sure it's easy to understand unless you have been through some form of it yourself.

Anon, 35

People are embarrassed to admit it, they need to know that there's nothing to be ashamed of. There is definitely not enough attention or awareness of it. It's an awful thing! I wanted to end it all so many times, I felt so alone.

Sam, 27

Unfortunately, there is very little awareness of PND in Ireland and for those who are aware, it is very misunderstood and even just called 'Baby Blues', which is definitely not the same thing. I had barely heard anything about it before I had it myself, the hospitals and antenatal classes should be under an obligation to inform people (both men and women) that it is a reality and very common, so that woman and their partners/families can see it coming and deal with it before it gets out of hand.

Anon, 32

I think people still think Post Natal Depression is all "in your head". I firmly believe that you can get away with a light dose if you get help and support from the start. It is a modern phenomenon that you are at home alone with your baby all day long with no support. Generations before us always lived together and help was always at hand. We are a very lonely generation. The Media is also to blame, putting pressure on women to get their shape back and be their old self again when really NOTHING is like it used to be any more. You have changed, your life has changed, your relationship has changed....

Sam

What advice would you give to other women suffering with Post Natal Depression?

Seek help as soon as you can, be it from family, friends, your public health nurse or your doctor. Don't leave it and hope it will go away. It's not your fault and there is no blame with this. You will only get better by being proactive about it no matter how afraid you are. Have hope in yourself and your ability to get better and even though it takes time you will get though the fog and be well and happy again.

Siobhan, 34

I would advise other women who are already suffering or suspect they are suffering from PND to get help as soon as you know something is not right, it won't go away by itself. Also don't feel guilty or ashamed....it is very common and will only get worse the longer it's left untreated. It doesn't always require medication, sometimes counseling/chatting is enough. If you are dismissed by someone you confide in, than turn to someone else, because it is a real illness and life is so much better when you get help.

Anon, 32

Don't be ashamed. Ask for help. Tell your friends and family, even bring them to the doctor with you if you want! Admit it! Get help. And there's nothing wrong with taking tablets to help you. You're not a failure in any way!! If I can do it you can too.

Sam, 27

I have always been out and about no matter what the weather was like and I think that that helped me. Also, instead of thinking about how every other mother has it easy and is on top of things and has lots of friends, I started talking to other mothers wherever I met them. It is a very lonely and isolating time but I realized that most of us are in the same boat. I joined a Mother and Toddler group and made great friends there and for a long time it was the highlight of my week to go there, have a cuppa and a chat. I also joined a gym with a crèche and it was great to get a bit of break, meet other grown- ups and just have something to do. Be out and about as much as you can. It's great for you and baby.

Christiane

Seek help. All the help you can get. Try anything and everything because there is no need to suffer, but it's so hard to see that when you are in the depths of it.

Anon, 35

My advice to other women would be to not be afraid to ask for help. Everyone loves to help! Don't be shy or feel guilty, if someone offers you a helping hand, take it. Don't let pride get in the way. And if you notice you are not feeling like your usual self, if you find it hard to get up or get motivated, speak to your GP about it.

Sam

POST NATAL DEPRESSION IRELAND
021 492 3162
www.pnd.ie
e mail support@pnd.ie

We hold monthly Support Meetings on the last Tuesday of the month at 8pm in Cork University Maternity Hospital, Wilton, Cork and encourage partners to attend the first night. We offer a support system for woman and their families going through Post Natal Depression.

Aside from our monthly support group we also run a support line where mums can talk to woman who have experience of PND and we have a dedicated website where mums can communicate with each other through the discussion section and the chat room. We are a voluntary organization and a registered charity.

We encourage women to contact their Public Health Nurse and
G.P.

*(Author's Note: I cannot recommend highly enough the book
"Recovering from Post Natal Depression," by Bernie Kealey
and Madge Fogarty, founders of PND Ireland. It offers a
world of hope and encouragement to women suffering from
post natal depression. Both of the authors suffered from PND
at some point in their lives but went on to make full recoveries
and set about setting up a service to help spread awareness and
to support PND sufferers. More information on the book can
be found at* www.pnd.ie*)*

Chapter Ten
HOME AND AWAY

A Working Mum

Guilt was a feeling I had few encounters with before becoming a mother. It was something that came upon me in my pre baby days, while lying in bed till noon nursing a sore head after a big night out. It would tap my shoulder, briefly reminding me that I was missing out on some of the finest hours of a beautiful day as I turned over and snoozed for another little while.

Nowadays however, GUILT is an emotion I am all too familiar with. It's always there in the background. Lingering, hanging around, and waiting for you to trip over it and some days it just knocks you right over.

Since becoming a mother, guilt is a feeling that becomes quite regular. You're always trying to do the best for your child and feel guilty if you can't give 110 %. Being a working mother, Guilt is a full-time lodger. I went back to work when my Son was eight months old and I can honestly say that it's one of the hardest things I've ever had to do. I realize that I was lucky to have been able to avail of some unpaid leave to be at home with my Son until then, but returning to work full time was heartbreaking.

The week before I was due back, I cried every day. I held my Son so tightly that last week hoping it would give me the strength to get through the following week. I thought of all the times I did the laundry and cleaned the house over the past eight months that I could maybe have skipped and had even more playtime and cuddles instead. Now, someone else was going to have all the enjoyment of him for the whole day while I went back to the big bad working world, far away from lazy mornings together in bed, breastfeeding on demand, gazing in wonder at his every move and singing happy silly songs.

At eight months, he had become so cute and fun and was learning new things every day. He was becoming more independent and anxious to explore his surroundings. He didn't need me so much anymore, as this new world he was discovering was so exciting. But I needed him...

How would I last eight hours without him?

For the first month back I did a four day week, which was great for both of us. It really eased us into things as I took Wednesday as my day off and it broke up the week nicely. He spent a day with each of his Nanas and two days with a very good friend of mine.

My first week back was such a novelty that I actually enjoyed it. For all the tears I had cried the previous week, when I woke on Monday morning and put on my suit, a switch went on and I moved into "Work Mode." I enjoyed catching up with the girls in the office, chit chat about this and that and having a whole hour to eat lunch by myself, not to mention a tea-break to boot!

As the weeks wore on and I returned to my regular five day week, it got a little harder. I missed my little man so much and felt pangs of guilt at handing him over to someone else every day. I almost resented hearing reports about any progresses he made while with his minders as it meant that I wasn't there and I had missed out.

He was reaching milestones while I was at the office trying to reach targets. It was so unfair. The worst was the day I arrived to collect him from the childminders to be informed that he'd cut his first tooth.

Why couldn't she let me find it myself? I had waited so long for it (nine months) and now I just felt like a useless mother as I wasn't the one to discover it. What if I missed his first steps? Chances are he was going to take them between the hours of nine and five, somewhere between Monday and Friday.

So many questions would go round in my head. Did he miss me when I wasn't there? Did he notice I was gone for so long? Did he remember I was his Mammy?

Often, in the evenings when I collected him, he would hardly glance at me, and while it was a little upsetting that he wasn't too bothered about me, I consoled myself with the fact that it confirmed how content he was with his minder. He was always very cheerful and never got upset by my arriving or leaving. My little boy was happy; it was me who had the separation anxiety.

Combining work & home life has been a struggle. Being organized is key and being organized is also something that I'm not always. Before returning to work, I cooked for weeks, stocking up the freezer with a few months supply of meals. When that ran out, it was never again replenished!
Some days though, I often plan a wonderfully stocked freezer full of homemade dishes in my head which keeps me going as I know I'll never have time to get around to it! Ironing is also a thing of the past, and if it's required, it's done on a need - only basis!

As time has moved on, working full time has just become the norm. I do hate being away from my child for so many hours a day but don't have a choice. My job doesn't offer part-time or flexi-time. I often feel that working mums are stuck between a rock and a hard place. I try to do my best at work and my best at home but my company like many other companies doesn't offer enough opportunities to their employees to help improve Work/Life Balance.

Another difficult issue for working mums is that of 'Climbing the Corporate Ladder'. While starting a family shouldn't mean the end of your career, there is more often than not an element of a glass ceiling within an organization when it comes to career advancement for working mothers.

Personally, I like working outside the home and while doing it five days a week isn't my ideal, at the moment its how it is. As time goes on, it has become easier to juggle work and home life. Once my son is happy, it's all that matters and I have learned to try not to beat myself up so much about it.

On the upside, weekends now have a whole new meaning. It's all about fun and family time together. It's what gets me through the week and keeps my spirits up on a tough day.

In my first year of parenting I've discovered that Guilt is something I'm always going to have to live with, it comes with the territory. In trying to do the best for your child, you will often feel that it is not enough. We sometimes set our standards too high. Nothing can be perfect all of the time and it's okay to take shortcuts.

Another thing I've learned is that life is short, it's for the living and we should try not to waste it on feelings of guilt and inadequacy. Our little ones grow up so fast and all we can do for them is our best.

Lisa O'Sullivan, Cork

Real Mams Talk About:
Returning To Work

It had always been my intention to go back to work, depending on contracts etc. plus, I'm a lecturer so the students would have arrived back on Sept 1st, which coincided nicely with the end of my mat leave. We probably could manage on just my husband's salary but like that I am extremely independent and love to get my own pay check, which is now permanent and pensionable. Plus I like my job, it's not too stressful most of the time and it keeps me organized. For a few weeks during my mat leave I did think it would be nice for me to stay at home, but I know that just wouldn't be for me. I'm not that person. Maybe if I had three or four children it would be different, but I'm happy with the way things are at the mo. Plus I'm going down to four days a week from Feb to sept, when we have fewer students, so I think that's a good balance for me.

I have a brilliant childminder, we don't have to get up insanely early and battle masses of traffic, I'm home with Izzy around 5.30 pm. I do have the odd pang of guilt, but I usually find that when I'm in work, I just get on with my job, I don't even go to Rollercoaster during work hours.......well maybe sometimes, during lunch!! Then in the evenings and weekends I've all the time in the world for Izzy.

Karen, 29

I chose to return to the workplace following the birth of my baby because of financial commitments e.g. mortgage. On returning to work I was devastated to have to leave my daughter for eight hours each day. I was quite emotional in the days leading up to my return date and couldn't believe how quickly the months had flown by. I found it really tough trying to balance the work and home life to the point of being emotionally and physically exhausted for the first two - three weeks. It was like starting a new job all over again on the first day back and I hated being there for the first few days as I knew I didn't have a choice in the matter because of the financial situation. It is slowly getting easier now and I have developed a routine so I don't feel as un-organized as I did the first week back.

Aisling, Dublin, Mam of One

I'm still on maternity leave, and I will be going back to work. It's a bit of a double edged sword as I don't really want to let her with anyone else but I also want to have some time away from her too. It's tough really, but it's okay with me as my hours aren't enormously long.

Jenny, Cork

I went back to work part-time for the reason that I am doing a job I really enjoy and see it as something I'd love to stay in for as long as I'm working. I feel that being a special needs teacher is a part of who I am and I didn't want to lose this. I am constantly learning new things that are applicable in my everyday life in my job so this was another thing I didn't want to lose out on. I did plan to have my daughter but I also planned to go back to work. I was open to the fact that I may not want to but when the time came I felt ready. Having said that, I am now doing part-time and could not do anymore and my interest in it has lessened. I still love it but am not as driven to move up in rank. Of course finance is another reason, but it was not the main reason.

Anonymous, 34, Roscommon

I went back to work after six months. I love my job very much but they are not baby friendly and during those early crèche days when my daughter was catching every illness going, they were not impressed that I had to take time off. We don't have a support network either, so we couldn't rely on anyone but ourselves. Thankfully that end has settled down and I hit the ground running so they can't complain. I feel sick with guilt every time I leave her. I'm leaving as she wakes and only get to see her for an hour and a half in the evening. On Saturday and Sunday, I make sure my time is hers. BUT... she is thriving in crèche. She has great social skills and loves all her little friends. She lights up when we come across kids anywhere, be it the supermarket, the park, etc... So I know that although it kills me leaving her she is in the best place possible.

Jennifer, 28, Meath

I had to go back to work. Ideally it would have been lovely to take the unpaid leave off to make it a year but it just wasn't viable. I felt shit about it. I didn't cry but I got very angry at everything and everyone. I managed to reduce my hours by eight a week but that was because the office moved whilst I was on maternity leave, and what had been a fifteen minute journey became a fifty minute commute. On the other hand though, I felt like I was going insane staying at home and was really looking forward to going back. My first lunch break was pure heaven. A whole hour to myself to eat! My son loves the creche though and it's done wonders for his confidence and development. Plus, I get the biggest smile and screech when I go and pick him up.

Kirsty, 29, Dublin

I was looking forward to going back to work as I got very bored with being at home and trying to find things to do. Maybe it's different when you have more than one baby as you're much busier. I loved being off in the summer but once it hit the winter months and my hubby was working long hours, I got very fed up being on my own a lot of the time. Working full time, five days a week, I am in much better form. I personally would go bonkers if I was to stay at home full time. I don't think it's good for anyone's mind!

Mam of One

I work full time. It was never a question of whether or not I would return to work. Financially I had to and apart from that I needed the break. I really admire stay at home mothers, I definitely could not do it. About three months after having my daughter I was ready to have a breakdown! My son is a very demanding toddler and he took all my energy without having a new baby as well.

Louise, 28, Cavan

I am just back to work two weeks now and have a seven month old baby boy. I commute from Tipp to Cork every day and have everything organized to a t! I could only do it with the fantastic help of my husband and an amazing childminder. I am also currently studying and sending in assignments for my CPA exams. It's all fun and games in our household! I find that organization is the key as well as having a hubby who really helps out in any way he possibly can. I needed to go back to work financially but also for my own sanity. We live in the back of beyond and I really love meeting people and the whole social aspect of work. Babs loves going to the childminders and is socializing with the best of them as the childminder minds two others also. When I am home I give my time and attention to my husband and babs and when I am at work I give 100 per cent so I don't have to take any work home with me. I fit the exam prep into study leave days and when all the family are asleep.

Niamh, 33, Tipperary

I work full time and my husband stays at home with the kids. It made sense for us as he had a medical reason to give up work and the construction industry was slowing down. I have a really good job which is flexible, pays for health care for the entire family and lets me work eight to four so I have a couple of hours with the kids in the evening. I don't worry about them one jot as they are with their Dad and he is every bit as good at looking after them as me.

A, 33, Dublin

Kathy's Story

I was a workaholic (was!!!!!) I thought nothing would ever interrupt my career as a teacher, I love my job. I was the one who said I would be back before maternity leave finished. Since the birth of my son though, work could not be further from my mind. I am dreading going back, I really don't want to leave him. He is four months old now which means I have two more months left with him. He does new things every day and I want to be there for everything.

For financial reasons I have to return to work full time. I have even considered giving up work and living on the basics but that is not practical, I am the main earner in the house and I pay the mortgage. And now in this economic climate and with pay cuts on the agenda things will be very tight indeed. Thank god I have good holidays.

I have looked into a crèche, it's proving to be a bit of a nightmare, I have heard so many bad stories of neglect and mistreatment of babies. I have found one place that I am sort of happy with, however, they don't open early enough for me to commute to Dublin and get to work on time, so it looks like I will become the late girl. I worry about how he will go for a nap without me there to sing him to sleep.

How will he feel when he sees the face of a stranger when he wakes up and not my face (I Always make a point of waking him with a smile) I worry that he will not get the same care that I give him as he won't be the only baby there. It also costs the same as my mortgage, how the hell I'm going to manage week to week I don't know. I discussed getting an Au pair with my husband as it is much cheaper but we decided that the Au pair may not have child care qualifications. Our house is small and there would be no privacy. A nanny is too expensive. I have interviewed a few childminders but none were suitable for a variety of reasons. I am so afraid of leaving the most precious thing in my life in the care of someone else.

I just wish I was on leave for at least a year or until he could talk and tell me if something was wrong. My husband rang me from work today saying that he was listening to the radio and they were discussing crèches. He said there were too many complaints and not one positive story. It's hard. It is so hard. I know I will cry when I have to leave him. I don't know how I'll cope. I don't know how he will cope. But I just keep thinking that I'm not the only one, I am not the first working mother and I won't be the last.

Tips on Returning to the Workplace from those already there...

Just think of the positives and know that you are doing the best for your child/children. Try and get into a routine and stick to it. Get organized, prepare dinners, bags, lunches and such the evening before so that there's no rushing in the morning. If possible, try and get more flexible hours. I have a very flexible & understanding boss and this helps. Make sure to get plenty of sleep and eat healthy. You will need all your energy! Don't worry about the housework, it will always be there. Do it at your convenience or hire a cleaner if it's financially possible in order to ease that burden.

Fiona, Dublin

Pick a creche that you are comfortable with so you aren't worried about the baby. Also, try and have a back-up plan in case your baby is sick. Something has got to give, you can't do it all. In my case, I don't have much time to meet friends anymore and my husband and I rarely go out alone together but I am trying to make more time for this!

Alison, Dublin

Be organized. Don't only think of the downside, you'll just get depressed. That being said though, only go back to work if you feel the benefits. If you spend all day pining for your babies, then they're where you need to be.

Lisa, Mam of Three, Sligo

The advice I would give to other women is to enjoy every moment of your maternity leave. It goes by way too fast. In the weeks leading up to going back to work, start getting up early each morning in order to allow your body clock time to adjust. Once back at work, try preparing the baby's dinners for the week ahead so you know your child is being fed what you are choosing. Plan a holiday or weekend away for a few months down the line so as to give yourself something to look forward to. Finally, take all the help that is offered your way as it will make things a lot easier to cope with.

Aisling, Dublin

Try not to get to get caught up in work. When you leave the office (or where ever you work) try and leave your work there, don't bring the stress home. Make the most of all the time you get with your family.

Nikki, Dublin

If there is any way possible that you can work part time or take parental leave and do a four day week - grab the opportunity! I think myself and my younger baby would have benefited hugely from me being at home a bit more.

Siobhan, Kildare

Suzanne's Story
I chose to become a stay at home mum when pregnant with my second daughter; mainly because it wasn't worth my while working and paying two creche fees as my wage just barely covered the cost! But there were other reasons too...

I went back to work after having my first daughter when she was only four and a half months old. I felt that I missed out on her first two years of life and I didn't want to do that to anymore of my children. I felt that by putting my kids in a creche all day, five days a week, someone else was rearing them and I didn't have kids only for someone else to rear them!

I love that I get to see my kids all day, every day. I can spend loads of time with them. I get to see all their first time happenings, like first steps, teeth, words etc... I know my kids and they know me. They get to know each other and can play together. I'm there when they need me. I can breastfeed for as long as I like with no pressure of work. There is no stress to get up in the morning, and rush around to get out to work on time. I get to do the house work during the week, so at weekends when daddy is home we can all spend loads of time together.

Things are very tight at the minute living on one income. We just have to cut back on luxuries and only buy the essentials. We don't have holidays, we don't go out at night time, we rarely get take-away and we only buy what we need and what we'll use in the weekly shopping. We don't buy new clothes just because we see something we like.

But we get by just fine. We do things with the kids that don't involve spending loads of money, like taking walks or going to the beach or to the playground. They don't notice any difference; all they want to do is have fun, no matter what it costs!

Yes, some days it can feel like you're doing the same thing every day. It can be a bit lonely without adult company all day. Living on one income is sometimes hard. But these cons don't go for everyday, and the pros outweigh them by a mile!

I'd advise other women that might be thinking about being a stay at home mum to just do it! Kids are only young once, they grow up so fast. They will be in school within five years and you can always return to work then if you want. Don't miss out on your kids first few special years of life!

Suzanne, Mam of two, Meath

Real Mams Talk about:
Staying Home

I went back to work after nine months of maternity leave. I never really wanted to go back and was unspeakably miserable during the week. To be honest, I don't think that anyone or any childcare would have been right for me even if it had been fine for my child. My son was in a creche and not sleeping or napping properly so when we collected him every day at five, he was shattered and we either had cranky time until bedtime or else he'd have to go straight to bed and then back up for another hour. We basically had no family time during the week. We took him out of creche and put him in a childminders care which was disastrous as she had lied to us and misrepresented herself. After a few spot-checks we took him out. We decided after doing the maths and realizing we could manage it, that I'd stay at home with him myself. I have never been happier.

Angela, Mam of One, Cork

For me there was no other choice. I wanted to be the one to raise my child and see them reach each milestone. There is so much growth in the first year and I didn't want to miss a thing! Being a mom is the best and hardest job in the world.

Denae, 23, Dublin

While pregnant with my first, I thought I'd be back at work in six months. I couldn't do it. And now, through my reading, I feel that if possible, children should be with a parent for a long time. Their needs are vast and cannot be given by a "carer" in the same way. That's my belief, there are many that disagree with me but in my bones I feel I'm right. Having it all is possible, but maybe not all at once. I may have to go back before youngest is two years for financial reasons, and I will be very sad but that's life.

Mairead

Some days I feel like I'm ready to be committed! I think most people being honest will say the same. And other days I feel like I've won the only lottery that matters.

Pamela

I just always wanted to be at home for my children. My mother was and I'm very grateful for that. Also I never liked working that much. I'm a work to live rather than a live to work person.

My husband and I had been married for almost ten years by the time our son arrived. We adopted him and after all that time and waiting I particularly wanted to make the most of the short time he'll be small and stay at home with him.

Gabi, 39, Dublin

All my life the only thing I knew for sure was that I wanted to be a mother. Somehow I just knew that when I had kids I would choose to stay at home with them. I just feel that these years are so precious and go by so quickly, I want to be there full time for them.

Anne, Mam of 2, Limerick

I chose to be a stay at home mum simply because I couldn't bear the thought of leaving my baby with anyone else. I had friends who were racing out the door in their eagerness to get back to the workforce, but the thought of leaving my child with a minder or in a creche made me uneasy and - if I am honest - insanely jealous! The thought of missing his milestones was too much for me to bear. My husband was more than happy with this arrangement as he too did not want our baby spending forty hours a week in a creche.

Helen, Mam of three, Cork

I was made redundant in my full-time job after maternity leave. I didn't want to leave my baby to work full-time, so I decided to stay at home with her. I feel it's important to be with her in these early years and I do plan to return to work once she starts school.

Lisa, 29, Dublin

I didn't really choose to be a stay at home mum, it just happened as I didn't have a career started at a young age. Now, after four babies , I have no choice but to be at home. Having said that though, I wouldn't have it any other way.

Kate, Mam of four, Sligo

Managing on One Income...
We are finding it hard in this financial climate. With my husband being self-employed it's hard to know what way we'll be from one week to the next. We are lucky to have some savings from when I worked full-time. We now shop in Lidl and Aldi, plus we do a lot of shopping when we are up north as it's cheaper.

Lisa, 29, Dublin

We are lucky. Because we'd been married nearly ten years before our son arrived, we were well settled and a bit older. We bought our house years ago so our mortgage is reasonably small. We had set up a small business in our house, a Montessori school, which has given me the opportunity to have an income without having to go out to work. When our son arrived I employed a teacher so I have not had to work but still have a small income. We are modest people, we don't spend a lot of money, we try to have an annual holiday - usually in Ireland - we have oldish cars and I don't spend a lot of money on clothes, shoes etc...

Gabi, 39, Dublin

We manage, just barely, but then, my partner is separated with two teenage boys that he pays maintenance for as well. Aside from that, he works hard. We are entitled to FIS (Family Income Supplement) and a medical card. As a couple who decided to have four more children, aside from the two older boys, we have to choose their after school activities carefully. I grew up with no brothers or sisters until I was thirteen years old, so it's extremely important to me to have family to lean on. Money can be an issue in our house and if you're giving up a large income to stay at home be prepared for the strain finances can take on a relationship.

Anonymous

To be honest, this isn't really a problem. My husband is doing well financially so its fine. I have always said though, that I'd rather live in a much smaller house and on a budget than go back to work before our daughter starts school.

Pamela

My husband was made redundant after Christmas so we are currently managing on no income which is difficult, but you just have to cut back on certain items in the shopping and buy only the necessities. When my husband was working he was in management and on a good salary so we managed well. Naturally, things changed when I gave up my job but it wasn't a huge shock, as it was something I had always spoken about doing if we were lucky enough to have children.

Trish, Mam of three, Limerick

We managed okay at first, but now that my husband is facing paycuts of 25%, it will be difficult. That being said though, we will not put our daughter into a creche in order for me to go back to work. We budget carefully, and will just be even more frugal!

Olwen, 27, Galway

The first thing to do is to move all your tax credits to your spouse. Also, there's a Home Carer Tax Credit if you are staying at home minding kids worth €900 p/a - be sure to claim this.
A factor in deciding to be a SAHD was the fact that we were paying €18,000 p/a on creche fees. When you consider how much of a second salary after taxes, etc ... was going on childcare there isn't that much of a drop in going from two incomes to one. What I find helpful is a spreadsheet detailing incomes and outgoing for each month (just the main things). When you have a better oversight of how your finances are and what bills are due it definitely makes planning ahead a whole lot easier.

Also, we've changed shopping habits to get more for our money. From a personal point of view, I'm less likely now to make impulse buys. Also I read a lot so I would have been used to buying at least one book a week. Now I use the library and hardly ever buy a new book - another bonus of this is that I'm more likely now to pick up books in the library that I may not have been willing to buy. So I have broadened my reading range also.

Eric, 33, Cork

I mind a little one four days a week which helps with the bills. We cut back on unnecessary spending and just manage on what we have.

Angela, Mam of One, Cork

I feel lucky to be a stay at home mom. My husband and I share a house with my brother-in-law which definitely helps enable me to stay at home with my daughter. Even if we weren't living with him, I think we would try to make it work. Breastfeeding is free! I also make my daughter's baby food and where you shop is a huge factor. Public transportation, cooking instead of going out (but do go out on occasion!) Also, when you're out shopping, remember to say to yourself, do I really need this?

Denae, 23, Dublin

Advice to New Parents
- Don't focus completely on the money aspect of things for your decision. Look at the whole work/life balance.
- Parent & Toddler Groups are great (although Mother & Toddler Group with lone Dad is a better description in my case!)..
- Get involved with something outside the home. I was part of the organizing committee that was responsible for a new primary school opening in our town last Sept. Also I'm involved with a group who are currently setting up an allotment garden scheme. If something on those scales seems a bit much then just sign up for a night course - it'll get you out of the house and you can learn a new

skill or two. I did a cookery course last Autumn - it got me out of the house and improved my skills in the kitchen.

- My wife brings the kids up to her folks place for a night every four to six weeks. I stay here, get a few DVDs and beers and have some quality time alone. I think having some downtime when you are looking after the kids all the time is very important.

Eric, 33, Cork

When you have a job you get regular breaks and a lunch break, you don't get those when you are a stay at home mom. So take a break... have your partner take the baby to the park or on a drive and hop into the bath, read a book, get your hair done, anything that helps you relax. If you are lacking in the sleep department, try to nap with your baby. Most of all, keep yourself busy! There are tons of groups, classes and other stay at home moms that want to meet up.

Denae, 23, Dublin

My advice would be, try and make a routine of the day. You don't always have to stick to it but it helps to pass the day and I find kids always behave better when they know what's coming next.

Also, try to get out every day for a short walk, even just to the local shop, seeing other grown ups even for five minutes is great. I found this a lot easier when I had only one child but I still try to get out most days now. Finally - and I should take my own advise on this! - if you make the decision to stay at home, be proud of it. Don't feel the need to make excuses as to why you do.

Anne, Mam of two, Limerick

Make sure money isn't going to be a big problem! But first, to put the money issue in perspective, ask yourself how badly you want to be raising your children yourself, rather than having a childminder or nanny doing the most important parts of your job.

Anonymous

If you want to do it and can afford it then do. It's a good life and the best job ever. Do get out and about. Go to parent and baby groups, go visiting, make friends with other stay at home parents.   Enjoy the moment. Don't always be rushing to get things done.

Gabi, 39, Dublin

It will take a while to develop your new identity and to strike the right balance. Often, although you are busy, you're moving at a much slower and less controllable pace than in other work-places. Also, during the hard moments, try to stay focused on the reasons you chose to stay at home with your kids.

Grainne, 32, Dublin

Patience.... patience and more patience. Don't lose your contact with friends who don't have kids. One day they will need you just as much as you need them now, they keep you informed of the life that doesn't have children in it, i.e what's the office gossip, what's happened on the night the girls went out and you couldn't make it because you had no babysitter...

Michelle, Mam of two

Take it as it comes. Get out of the house and join a baby/toddler group. Make time for yourself. Don't wear trackie bottoms and tie back your hair everyday or you'll lose all your self esteem. Remember that nobody is perfect.

Pamela

If you can afford to do it then go for it! I think it gives your children a great start in life and who could be better to bring them up than their mammies? I know it is not for everyone but I truly don't think you would regret it. They are small for such a short time and I personally would hate to look back in twenty years time and think that I was never there for them because I was always at work. As I said before, I am in a lucky position to be able to do it even though financially we struggle. I don't care that we are scraping by though as I know that no amount of money would bring back their precious early years.

Helen, Mam of three, Cork

Chapter Eleven
GUILT

An Exercise in Guilt

Alex is shouting. He might be two and a half but he knows what he wants. It's nine am and it's time for his bottle of milk. I climb out of unconsciousness, roll off the bed and trundle down the stairs in just a pair of boxers.

I grab the liter of milk from the fridge and manage to get it everywhere – except into the damn bottle. Behind me, I'm aware of the woman next door – I don't even know her name – walking past the window with her three year old daughter. Their car is parked outside. I'm sure she saw me. I don't care.

Back upstairs, Alex takes the bottle with one hand and with the other, points to the pieces of a Thomas the Tank Engine jigsaw on the floor. I throw them in to the cot, with a Barney book for good measure.

His mother started her day an hour ago - she is in work. I have twenty minutes before mine begins. That's how long Alex will play with his toys before he wants out of his cot.

I climb back into bed. It's my own fault. I stayed up late last night playing computer games, thinking I was off today. I am not off though, I am minding Alex. I vow to go to bed earlier tonight and I start to doze, and dream about work.

Alex's voice is reaching for me again – a long high-pitched "aaah". He is not upset, yet. I pick him up and bring him into bed with me. Maybe he will go to sleep here? He never does. This morning is no exception. He crawls from the blanket beside me, onto my face and reaches up for the drink of water on the shelf above. The smell of urine and soggy nappies fills my nostrils. I'm awake now.

Downstairs, this time with a dressing gown on, I'm trying to change Alex's nappy. He is grinning, and kicking his legs in the air. I wipe his bum, trying (and failing) to not get shit on my fingers. I stick the tapes of the nappy together and look down. He has a full set of teeth, blue eyes and what looks like a receding hairline. I see my Dad, doing this. I cringe. I think of the words of JM Barie. "All of this has happened before, and all of this will happen again."

Alex and I are back upstairs. All I can see are towels. I'm deep in the hot press looking for a jumper – any jumper. Now is not the time for being fashionable. The stairs are waiting for Alex, ready to snap him up in their jaws and swallow him down to the hard wooden floors below. This is a flash point. A few weeks ago, I caught Alex swinging out of the stair-gate, at the top of the stairs. I went to grab his arm. He looked at me. And let go of the gate. "Bye Daddy". Then he fell.

Time did not slow down. I sped up and I jumped three steps at a time. There was no need. Alex wasn't even hurt. He cried for thirty seconds, pointing accusingly at the stairs. Then he ran into the sitting room looking for his "Barney book". But my hand was shaking. The stairs had taken a taste. I should have been watching.

My conscience was though. It's an observer. It documents all my fuckups and successes with Alex, for me to replay in bed each night. I've stayed up late watching the one where he stood up after falling down the stairs.

Alex eats warm crushed Weetabix for breakfast – or at least most mornings he does. "No Daddy," he shouts, as I sit down to my breakfast (strong sweet coffee). He is holding the bowl of Weetabix up the air at an awkward angle. I watch in growing frustration as the cereal drips down his jumper, and onto the floor. "A bar," he demands and he points at the press where the Smarties are kept.

"God damn it Alex!". It was cute the first morning he did this, not the tenth. I feel bad for shouting though and I consider giving him a packet. No one will know.

Minding Alex is an exercise in guilt. Is this the memory he is going to pull out of the fog of childhood when he is older – me shouting at him over spilt Weetabix and Smarties? I decide against the giving him a packet. Instead I look for cloth to clean up the Weetabix with, before they dry.

Ten minutes have gone by and I am shouting. "Alex!" He ignores me. He is using the door of the washing machine to climb up and reach for the switch on the kettle. Images of scars and blisters bubble before me. The scars and blisters of a boy I half-knew, his face ruined from a hot iron that he pulled on top of himself. I yank Alex off the machine. He cries in frustration. "That's bold!" I shout. I feel my conscience watching, taking notes.

I blame the house. It's too small for the two of us. I can see him breaking things, breaking himself. We – I – need to get out. The military operation begins. I gather the baby essentials: nappies, check; wipes, check; drinks, check; snack, check. Baby?

Let's go to the balls." He squeals, runs in a circle and starts laughing. There's that guilt again. "Balls" is his word for the local baby gym. "Balls" is baby-talk. I hear my granny's voice, "They'll never learn to speak properly if the parents are at it too."

"It's better than shouting at a two year old," I reason. But it's hard to win an argument with a dead person. Outside, the sun is pressing down hard on the estate. And it's quiet. Most people are at work. Are they dozing in front of their keyboards thinking about home? I press the button on the car key. Alex runs around to the driver's seat. He opens the door and hops in. Traffic is not one of his concerns. Nor are my shouts at him to stop. "What do you think you are doing?" I'm sweating now. He bangs the horn and grins. "Beep, beep!"

I eventually manage to strap Alex in his car-seat, start the car and turn up the radio. He's up. He's fed. He's watered. I'm doing a good job. Then, halfway down the road, I see him in the rear view mirror. He has one arm half out of his car seat and the other is reaching down for the open button. I shout at him to stop and slam on the brakes. He looks surprised.

We're at the Playzone, that obstacle course for babies. Slides, ramps, ball-pits, tunnels, climbing ropes – they're all present. And they are all padded. Someone has drawn animals on the walls. The place makes a rave look muted. I like it here. There is nothing for Alex to break and I don't have to clean up. Before Alex I was born I was barely aware places like this existed.

During the weekend, the Playzone is busy. It is as busy and as loud as any nightclub. Today, there are four or five groups of women in tracksuits sitting at the coffee tables near the baby gyms. They are drinking tea and chatting. Several men are here too. They are standing by themselves or following their kids around. My role is clear and I start following Alex.

He climbs inside the door of the larger baby gym and then he pulls himself up the padded steps onto the second floor. Already, I can see he is having second thoughts. His face is turning red and it is only a matter of time before –"Daddy!" he screams.

Beside me, a man is telling his daughter to "Go on" and pointing at the slide. I notice he's unshaven too. We avoid each other's eyes. Alex is bawling now. People are looking over, so I go in after him. He sees me and smiles. I am the hero in his adventure gone awry.

After an hour of this, we leave. At home, Alex is clearly inspired by the Playzone. He starts climbing on top of the washing machine, the stairs and even the toilet. I find myself shouting at him again. I put him into his cot for a nap. It's more for my sake than his. After a few minutes, silence enters the house. It takes something heavy off me. The dishwasher is still full and the wash basket overflowing. I make a cup of tea and sit down. This isn't that hard.

Alex is still asleep when my mate Jack calls up. I have known Jack for about ten years. He is in the middle of buying a house with his girlfriend. "How's Alex?" he says. Jack's balding head looks like it's been bolted down onto his body – as if God forgot to include a neck. He is here to see how to download music off the internet. Upstairs, as the computer boots up I tell Jack to keep it down. "We don't want to wake Alex," I say.

A roar erupts from the next room. Alex is awake and hot with anger. His roars are burning my ears. The redness of his cheeks matches the anger in his voice. His little fingers scratch my hands. He pushes me away. After five minutes of this, Jack turns to me and says "Does he ever stop?" I look at him for a second more than is polite. Jack wants four or five kids of his own.

I bribe Alex to stop with a biscuit and sit him on my lap. He starts banging the keyboard. Jack and I give up and go downstairs, where he asks if he can play my copy of Grand Theft Auto IV. I want to play it too, so I open the back door for Alex to go outside. Violent computer games don't interest him (yet).

Jack plays the game for a minute, before Alex runs in with holding a lump of grass. "That's dirty," he tells us. Then, Alex picks up a baby wipe off the ground and starts cleaning Jack's t-shirt.

I hope it's not a dirty one, one I used to change his nappy with. I feel good though. If Jack gets his way, he will know this soon.

After Jack leaves, I give Alex something to eat. He spills most of the sausages and beans onto the floor. We go for a walk to see the ducks. The "Wah Wahs", he calls them. Down at the canal, a mother duck is swimming with three ducklings. There were six here a few days ago. I wonder what happened to the other three.

Alex wanders a little closer to the edge of the canal. I can feel that stairs, that kettle, that car. And I reach for his arm.

The more I get to know Alex, the more I want to keep life from him. This is my problem. How will he learn how to keep the shit off his fingers with me in the way? I know I have plenty of time, but I haven't earned my parenting credentials. I should be frog marched out of the playground. Alex is already reaching away from me, and I am only figuring out how to reach for him.

A couple are sitting in a field nearby. They look relaxed and I envy them. That field looks more familiar. It looks more...I lose my train of thought. Someone small is tugging on my arm. "Yellow," Alex says and he points at the slide. He's right. It is yellow.

In the playground, Alex runs off shouting and pointing at the other kids, the birds, and dirty banana on the ground. I sit down on a bench by myself and look at my watch. He sees me, runs over laughing and gives me a hug. Surprised, I suddenly feel good about bringing him here.

This is what I am fighting my mistakes with. I am placing ordinary things down for Alex to see. I am armed with the ducks, the balls and the Playground and a notion, a notion that he will take one of these things, dust if off and use it when his own conscience cries out.

But I've already made mistakes. What if he carries them with him too?

Over at one of the slides a blond man in his thirties is playing with three kids. He is unshaven, wearing runners and a tracksuit. Alex gets on a wooden see-saw with one of the boys. "Cillian, go easy," the man tells the boy.

Alex and Cillian start bouncing up and down. Cillian is bigger than Alex and he is sending him higher and higher. "How old is he?" the man asks me. I visualize Alex launching into the air and landing on the ground in a broken mess. "Two and a half," I say. "Are they all yours?"

I put hand on Alex's back to steady him. The man nods and laughs.

"They keep you busy," I add. Then not being able to think of anything else to say, I pick up Alex and tell him it's time to go. He starts to cry.

I tell him, "We'll come again".

By Bryan Collins

Real Mams Talk About:
Bad Mammy Moments

Well, on two occasions I accidentally drove to my mum's house twenty minutes away with my son in his car seat and the straps open. I had completely forgotten to close them! I was in the horrors for weeks after.

Emma, 29, Cork

I find that plonking him in his chair in front of "Bear in The Big Blue House" is a great help in the mornings so that I can shower, clean up, eat, etc... His granny would not be impressed. So what! I can't entertain him all the time.

Fiona, 28, Kildare

When my daughter was six days old I was carrying her out of the bedroom in her moses basket. I put the two handles in one hand to open the door and one of the handles slipped out of my hand which tipped the basket and made her fall on the floor, smack on her forehead. I cried longer than her! She was fine, just a nice big bump on her forehead. Bad Mommy!!!

Chris, 31, Cork

With my first, I was a smoker. Although I only ever had one or two a week while I was pregnant, as soon as I had stopped breast feeding, I was back on them as bad as ever. There were times that he would be screaming and nothing I did would help, so I would leave him cry and go have three minutes "sanity" and a ciggie. I once left my nine month old daughter with my five year old son so I could get the washing in, and of course, she toppled over and bumped her head. Feeling terribly guilty, but not wanting to admit it, I gave out to my son for not minding her properly. That is probably the worst thing that I have done. I felt soooo bad afterwards that I explained it all to him and assured him that it was all my fault and that I realized I cannot expect a five year old to be able to mind a baby!

Christine, 29, Wicklow

I fed my baby from Jars...there I've said it loud and proud, and you know what? She is GREAT! She is running around at eleven months old and it has done her no harm. Monday – Friday, she has home cooked food in crèche. But on the weekends, breakfast and tea are homemade and dinner is from a jar. She gets all excited when she sees me spoon a lumpy concoction into the bowl. I have a baby, a relationship and a career. My time is too precious to be tied to a cooker mashing and peeling!

Jennifer, 28, Meath

In general I'm a very safety conscience and hygiene obsessive, but when I was starting to wean my daughter on to solids, I would be heating her purees in the microwave and she would be wailing to be lifted and instead of leaving her safely crying for a few minutes I would carry her while making her food. Then one day, I dropped the boiling hot puree onto the counter and some of it splashed onto her. I got it off before it burnt her but she felt it and really sobbed so I have never done it again. She is safer crying than near hot food or drink.

Ingrid, 29, Cavan

My son was around two months old and I had laid him naked in the middle of our bed to have a little kick. I turned my back for literally two seconds and I heard a "thump." I thought something had fallen off his changing table so my gaze went there first. When I realized nothing there had fallen, I turned to the bed and yep, there he was , on the floor beside the bed, naked and letting out a big scream. My heart was in my mouth as I lifted him up. He was fine and stopped crying as soon as he was in my arms, but I got some fright! How he managed to get from the middle of the bed to the floor in two seconds amazes me still!

Kim, 22, Dublin

Yeah, I've done the whole clipping his fingertip along with his nail and the five hours in a dirty nappy. I've probably given him calpol a couple of times when he doesn't really need it. I screamed at a wall once because I was so frustrated. Harry had been crying all day and I hadn't eaten. He was very quiet after that. Before Christmas, he was grumpy and wouldn't eat. I started blaming the creche for spoiling him with rusks. So I said "Harry, you're not having any rusks or dessert until you eat your dinner!" I was angry because I just thought he wanted a rusk. Anyway, after holding the spoon in front of his lips solidly for two minutes to try and get him to open his mouth and him crying and throwing his head back, I just said, "right, fine, but no rusk!" I took him out of his highchair and sat on the floor with him to calm him down and he felt very hot. I took his temperature and it was forty degrees! I was so upset at myself. It was still the same the next day so we went to the doctor. It turned out he had tonsillitis. No wonder the poor little mite didn't want to eat. That was my worst one...so far!

Kirsty, 29, Dublin

There have definitely been more than a few bumps when my back was turned, but there has also been the leaving him in a shop and walking out for a minute because I forgot that he was with me, Oh and let's not forget the time that I dropped him out to my sister but forgot to tell her that he was there. She rang me an hour after I left and inquired as to why I hadn't informed her that the baby was there. She thought that I had brought him with me, but he had been asleep in the cot. She was about to leave for town when she heard him whimper in the room...Whoops :(

Laura, 23, Tipperary

My worst bad mummy moment was when I had a flu I couldn't shake. So I made an appointment with the gp and decided to bring my son too as he had a very slight cough, the fact of the matter being that I wouldn't have brought him to the doctor only for the fact that I was sick myself. When discussing it with the doctor, it was broken to me that he had asthma. So much for my mother knows best belief. I hadn't a clue. My poor baby has been on an inhaler since.

Luke's Mom, Cork

Chapter Twelve
FUTURE MUSINGS...

The Mama Bear

Just the other morning, I was doing my usual routine of procrastination before setting down to write, when I came across a new friend's photos on Facebook. Nothing out of the ordinary mind you, just a typical album of family photos. No starving children or abandoned animals, just loads of shots documenting the first year of her older son's life.

As her little boy is three now and I've only known her since the birth of her second baby, these pics were new to me. They showed me a side of this woman I've never seen before.

Of the mothers I know, she is the capable one. The one who's done this mothering lark before and who seems to have it all together. She is the one whose eyes say "I've been here before" and who's hands know what they're doing. She is the one whose lap was made for curling up in and whose arms are filled with strength and comfort. She has the husband, the kids, the house, the dog... Her life, from my perspective at least, seems solid.

When I looked at her pictures though, I saw another side.

I saw a woman, heavily pregnant on her first baby, her dark eyes filled with hope; looking out at the camera with the smallest of smiles, as if to say, "Is this really happening?"

I saw a new mother, her baby clinging to her chest for warmth and security, her eyes still tired from the birth but her entire person suddenly alert and filled with a new life's purpose.

I saw the mama bear who would die for her cub before letting any harm befall him.

I saw her oldest boy brand new again, looking so much like his younger brother and yet different enough that you knew it wasn't.

I saw a family in progress and a mother in the making.

I saw the past that had shaped the present I know.

But most of all, I saw a side of my friend that I'd never seen before. One that had the tears filling my eyes and rolling down my cheeks. It was a softer more uncertain side that looked out and grabbed at your heart and made me want to pull her into my lap and wrap my arms around her, offering her what strength and comfort I have. And when she was wrapped up safe and snug I would stroke her hair and tell her stories of the future.

About the most capable mother I know.

Real Mams Talk About: Hopes and Dreams for my Baby's Future
I hope that they remain happy, healthy and confident. I think that these are three basic human rights and that if you have them; you can go on from there.

I want them to enjoy school, to enjoy the experience of learning and hopefully, continue on to college. I want them to be confident in themselves and expect others to treat them with respect and to have the ability to take a stand if this doesn't happen. I never had this confidence in myself. It took me a long, long time to get it.

You hear every day about the people who slipped through the system and left school with basic reading and writing skills. Well, I'm the maths equivalent of that. I remember being called up to the blackboard in 5th or 6th year and asked to work out a maths equation. I may as well have been asked to translate a page of Mandarin.

All I was taught that day by the teacher, a woman who was probably only a few years older than I was at the time, was to feel stupid, embarrassed and ashamed - all in front of 30 of my contemporaries. I'm sure if she were to meet me on the street today, she wouldn't know me, let alone remember that day. But I've never forgotten it.

I look at my 21 year old sister today and the confidence she has that I've only managed to achieve for myself in my very late twenties. Yes, confidence in yourself is so important.

I hope that my children find a job that they love and are good at. I hope that they travel before settling down. I hope that their first serious relationship does not run for more than a year. (Oh God, is there a "Mother in Law from Hell" in training here??)

I fear them getting hurt, both physically and emotionally. I fear them falling foul to the good things in life, so much so that they don't know when to stop. I fear them not having a good time.

I want them to know the difference between right and wrong and accept the consequences of both. I want them to value family; especially each other. I want them to have respect for others and themselves and have the confidence and ability to take a stand for what they believe in. It is my strongest hope though, that they feel able to talk to their parents about anything and that they would be comfortable coming to us with their problems, big and small.

Their Daddy is definitely the brains of the outfit so naturally enough, it would be great if the boys (and future children) followed suit. I would, however, not like them to inherit his sense of time! Different. Planet. Altogether.

I think I'd like them to have my sense of humor but not my temperament.

Whew! Reading back on that I realize I'm not asking for much!!!

Gwen, Kildare

I want my baby to have good family values. I want her to appreciate the value of money and of life. We have set up investment accounts for her to ensure if anything happened to us that she would be looked after. As for qualities, if she gets her father's brains and my looks she will be sorted!!!! (kidding!)

Leanne, 26, Donegal

I worry about what kind of world he's going to grow up in. It's getting harder and harder to survive with hate and violence everywhere, but then, I think our parents must have felt like this with us. I just want him to be happy. Really! I've spent most of my adult life looking for something and there's a saying that goes something like not having to travel to far and dusty lands to seek what you desire, you should be able to find it where you are (very loose explanation.) I want to teach him to happy and grateful with what he has here. Instill good family values and good manners in him, encourage and support him in whatever he chooses. I hope he gets my husbands sense of calm and reason but a little of my feistiness too. I hope he doesn't get too much of my temper though, otherwise we're buggered.

Kirsty, 28, Dublin

God, I have to say that even at this early stage I worry about them going out as teenagers and drink and drugs and all that goes with it. I wonder how I am going to instill in them that drugs are wrong, wrong, wrong, that cannabis use, no matter what you hear is dangerous and that getting drunk out of your face is not cool. Basically, I want to lock them in their bedrooms!

I think getting them involved in stuff is the way to do it. I am a firm believer in the benefits of sport; if they love something like Gaelic football or soccer, and they love that more than they want to go and get drunk, well then, you're halfway there. But that has to be instilled in them from an early age, God love our little lad, if you ask him who he follows, he'll immediately shout Liverpool and the Dubs. He's really getting into the football now, so if he can keep it up, I reckon it'll stand him in good stead.

I want them to be mannerly and thoughtful adults. My God if I ever hear of either of them bullying anyone in school, they'll know all about it. You hear so much about kids being distraught because they are being bullied, I would absolutely kill them if they were mean to another child. I would be so upset if anyone did it to mine.

As for inherited qualities...Probably my husband's ability to collect friends wherever he goes, and my ability to be passionate about whatever they choose to be passionate about - it's the only way to live!!

Anon, 33, Dublin

I want them to be safe, secure and happy and to know that they are very much loved. I really want them to be educated, and feel that university is not a choice but a given for them all. I hope they are confident, strong and secure like their dad and not worried about what other people think so much like me. I hope that their world is safe and exciting and that they travel and experience life to the full while knowing they can always come home.

Amber, 36

I want my babies to do what every it is that makes them happy. I would like them to learn that they do not have to conform to what society says is the "right" way. I hope they have my husband's patience, and my organization skills. I sincerely hope they do not inherit my mood swings and impatience. Whatever happens, as long as they are happy, I don't mind what they do.

Christine, 29, Wicklow

I hope my daughter will see me as a friend as well as her mam and as someone she can talk to about anything. I want her to have a happy and healthy life and not get involved with the wrong crowds, mixed up with drugs or into underage drinking.

I am a big animal lover and I hope that she will have respect for animals and never be cruel to them; although I don't think I have to worry on this as she is animal mad already!

I believe that you should earn everything you get in life and therefore have more respect for it. So I would like my daughter to do small tasks, like tidying her room for pocket money and when she is older, to save up for things like computer games or cars.

I worry about the kind of world my little girl will grow up in. Every day there are reports of murders and violence and sometimes they don't even make it to the front page meaning the value of life is not as important as it once was.

I hope that she will do her best in school or college but I will also support her 100% in whatever path in life she chooses to take.

My husband is a very hard worker which I admire but I also believe it's important to take time out and have fun and this will be something I hope that I hope my daughter will grow up with. I am a big worrier and get myself very stressed about the silliest of things. I will try not to let her see me like this so that she will be a confident young girl with no worries.

Ingrid, 29, Cavan

No major fears as we have strong religious beliefs that deal with those issues. I hope that the children grow up as well adjusted, productive people who are happy in their own skins and contribute to other people's happiness. Hopefully, they don't inherit my quick temper (too late there I think! My bad example!) We would probably be happy to see them grow up with a similar work ethic to us which would include voluntary work. Our emphasis would be on being happy and full-filled, not material things.

Samantha

Ultimately, all I want is for my baby to be happy and healthy. I would like her to have some manners, and not to be spoiled beyond belief. I think it's inevitable that she will end up being a bit of a nerd (we both are) and I'm okay with that. I'd like her to have our weird sense of humor I just want her to be safe.

Jenny, Cork

I hope my baby has confidence, not just in the social sense but confidence and strength enough to do whatever he wants with his life, even if that means not conforming or even if he has to go against what I want for him. I want the best for him and I admit I would rather he got a good education and career somewhere down the line but I don't want to become that kind of cliche middle class parent who starts off saying once he has his health, thats good enough - then ten years later is hung up on which private school will take him and feels he must be a doctor or solicitor and nothing else is good enough.

I want him to have a sense of morality and the ability to question everything - not just be a sheep.

As for inheriting qualities, both me and my husband are very honest. Ronan can be honest to a fault, really blunt whereas I am probably a bit more sensitive and I suppose can be false depending on the social situation, but mostly where it matters I am honest and don't understand people who lie or exaggerate or never admit failure. I hope my baby inherits these qualities, ideally somewhere in between the two of us.

I can lack drive and ambition sometimes which frustrates me, whereas my husband is very driven and can be too competitive sometimes. I hope my baby doesn't follow either or us and finds a happy medium.

Laura, Cork

My biggest hope for my beautiful baby girl is to be happy in her own skin, whatever she decides to do in her life. I hope she is independent, strong and has the courage to do and go for things in life that I never did. I hope she stands up for herself but not aggressively, assertively. We have no control over how the world is going to be in the future but I hope I give her a happy, loving childhood so that she will always have good memories of her home life when she is all grown up. As for qualities she inherits from hubby and I... Hmm...

From hubby - strong personality, good hair, long legs (mine are awful) and the ability to make money. From me, I'd like her to have creativity, brains, beauty, good figure (I did have one once!) kindness, honesty, patience and love. Of course she will inherit some qualities or not that are not so nice like a bad temper, no patience, arrogance, the use of bad language (from daddy) and being too quiet for her own good (from mammy).

Amanda, 32, Limerick

I want her to be happy in herself, to never feel she has to live up to some stupid expectation of someone else. I hope she will be her own person and know her own mind, be independent, and get a good job as a primary school teacher in a small country school (ha ha ha.) I hope she'll be able to talk to me and with me, I don't really have that relationship with my mom, but I hope to with my own daughter. I hope she'll be kind and optimistic. I hope she won't have to worry about things and I obviously hope she has a long and happy life. Oh and I hope she'll have siblings....

Karen, 29

I want my kids to have manners, please and thank you go a long way. I am really pushing it on Philip to use his Please and thank you. I hate cheeky kids with no manners! I want them to appreciate things and treat others with respect.

I hope my son does not inherit the whole "let the women do it all" thing! I hope he learns to be more patient and less aggressive than their father.

I hope they are confident individuals not afraid to speak their mind and stand up for themselves. I hate that I have no back bone and find it very hard to fight my corner, I let people walk all over me much to my husband's annoyance. I want them to be happy and to see beyond the end of their own noses, not to be selfish.

Louise, 28, Cavan

Wow! That's a biggie! Well I hope my girls grow up to love me and each other like I love them. I hope they are happy and know how much they mean to me. I want them to be good, honest people. Moral.

I know the world's probably going to be in an even worse state when they grow up, it scares me to think about it. I hope they don't get involved in drugs etc...

I hope they never get bullied in school like I was and that they have loads of friends.

I hope they understand that I left their dad because I felt we deserved better than to be treated like that. I don't want them growing up thinking that it's okay for men to treat women like that and get away with it.

I want them to be strong women like I am trying to be. I am only 26 and trying to be strong for the three of us!

I hope they still love me even though I left their dad.

I hope they are strong, successful, respectful and respected women.

I hope they don't have a temper like mine and grow to be a bit less of a stress head than I am.

God! I could go on and on but I won't! I can barely type for the tears...

I just want them to know how much they are loved, that alone will get you through anything.... x

Samantha, 26

Resources:

Parenting Websites:
Great places to go to get general information as well as plenty of advice and support on all aspects of parenting!
www.rollercoaster.ie
www.magicmum.ie
www.mumstown.ie
www.babywearingireland.com
www.attachmentparentingireland.eu/ireland
www.dad.ie
www.drjaygordon.com
www.drsears.com

Parenting and Childbirth Associations
Cuidiu (The Irish Childbirth Trust)
Web: www.cuidiu.com
Phone: 01 872 4501

La Leche League Ireland
A voluntary organization that provides support and information to breastfeeding mothers.
Web: www.lalecheleagueireland.com
Email: leader@lalecheleagueireland.com

Association of Lactation Consultants in Ireland
Web: www.alcireland.ie

Friends of Breastfeeding
Friends of Breastfeeding is a voluntary organization that aims to offer support and information to breastfeeding mothers and to foster a positive breastfeeding culture in Ireland.
Web: www.friendsofbreastfeeding.ie

The Breastway
Online support and advice for breastfeeding mothers in Ireland.
Web: www.thebreastway.com

Jack Newman Dot Com
Incredible website offering accurate and up to date information and support on breastfeeding by one of the world's foremost experts, Dr. Jack Newman
Web: www.drjacknewman.com

Kellymom
Breastfeeding support and information
Web: www.kellymom.com

Gentle Birth: Hypnosis for Pregnancy and Birth
www.gentlebirth.ie
www.birthingmamas.ie

The Homebirth Association of Ireland
A voluntary organization that provides information to women interested in having a home birth in Ireland.
Web: www.home birth.ie
Email: enquiries@home birth.ie

Association of Irish Doulas
Web: www.doula.ie

Doula Ireland
Web: www.doulaireland.com

Caesarian and VBAC Support
Web: www.ican-online.org
Web: www.informedbirthireland.com
Web: www.vbac.com
Web: www.vbacfacts.com

Cosleeping dot org
Offering easy access to the best information sites on Co sleeping
Web: www.cosleeping.org

The Irish Multiple Births Association (IMBA)
IMBA is a voluntary association which provides information and support to expectant parents and families of multiples.
Web: www.imba.ie
Email: info@imba.ie
Phone: 01 874 9056

Irish Premature Babies
A voluntary organization set up by parents who have had premature babies They offer support and information to parents of preterm babies.
Web: www.irishprematurebabies.com

Single Parent Support
www.gingerbread.ie
www.solo.ie
www.treoir.ie

Post Natal Depression Ireland
POST NATAL DEPRESSION IRELAND
Web: www.pnd.ie
e-mail: support@pnd.ie

Phone: 021 492 3162
We hold monthly Support Meetings on the last Tuesday of the month at 8:00pm in Cork University Maternity Hospital, Wilton, Cork and encourage partners to attend the first night. We offer a support system for woman and their families going through Post Natal Depression.

Aside from our monthly support group we also run a support line where mums can talk to woman who have experience of PND and we have a dedicated website where mums can communicate with each other through the discussion section and the chat room. We are a voluntary organization and a registered charity.

We encourage women to contact their Public Health Nurse and G.P.

(Author's Note: I cannot recommend highly enough the book "Recovering from Post Natal Depression," by Bernie Kealey and Madge Fogarty, founders of PND Ireland. It offers a world of hope and encouragement to women suffering from post natal depression. Both of the authors suffered from PND at some point in their lives but went on to make full recoveries and set about setting up a service to help spread awareness and to support PND sufferers. More information on the book can be found at www.pnd.ie)

Parentline
Help line for parents and Guardians. They also teach several parenting courses.
Web: www.parentline.ic
Email: info@parentline.ie
Phone: 1890 927 277

The Irish Sudden Infant Death Association
ISIDA offers support and information to families who have suffered the loss of an infant or young child.
Web: www.isida.ie
phone: 1850: 391 391

Miscarriage Association of Ireland
Voluntary organization which aims to offer support and information to parents who have suffered pregnancy loss.
Web: www.miscarriage.ie

AIMS Ireland
A consumer led voluntary organization which aims to highlight normal birth and campaign for mother and baby friendly birth practices in Ireland.
Web: www.aimsireland.com

The World Health Organization
Web: www.who.int/en

Health Service Executive
Web: www.hse.ie

ABOUT THE AUTHOR

MARIA MOULTON is the mother of two perfect little girls who have slept through the night since the day they were born and have never given their parents a moment of trouble since. She is in fabulous shape and never has a hair out of place. Her personal style has been described as "effortless" and her home, "immaculate." She is up to date on current affairs and regularly throws elegant soirees for visiting dignitaries.

Her blog can be found at **www.mammydiaries.blogspot.com**